**Disorders of Human Communication 5**

Edited by G.E. Arnold, F. Winckel, B.D. Wyke

M. Hirano
# Clinical Examination
# of Voice

**Springer-Verlag  Wien New York**

Minoru Hirano, M.D.

Professor and Chairman, Department of Otolaryngology, Kurume University, Kurume, Japan

With 36 Figures

ISSN 0173-170X
ISBN 3-211-81659-3 Springer-Verlag Wien-New York
ISBN 0-387-81659-3 Springer-Verlag New York-Wien

# Editors' Foreword

This volume is one in a series of monographs being issued under the general title of "Disorders of Human Communication". Each monograph deals in detail with a particular aspect of vocal communication and its disorders, and is written by internationally distinguished experts. Therefore, the series will provide an authoritative source of up-to-date scientific and clinical information relating to the whole field of normal and abnormal speech communication, and as such will succeed the earlier monumental work "Handbuch der Stimm- und Sprachheilkunde" by R. Luchsinger and G. E. Arnold (last issued in 1970). This series will prove invaluable for clinicians, teachers and research workers in phoniatrics and logopaedics, phonetics and linguistics, speech pathology, otolaryngology, neurology and neurosurgery, psychology and psychiatry, paediatrics and audiology. Several of the monographs will also be useful to voice and singing teachers, and to their pupils.

**G. E. Arnold,** Jackson, Miss.
**F. Winckel,** Berlin
**B. D. Wyke,** London

# Preface

In the field of otology and audiology, several techniques for the clinical examination of auditory function have been established and standardized. As a result of the standardization of these techniques, it is possible to compare the auditory function of different subjects examined at different places and/or different occasions and to monitor the results of treatments in a reliable manner. With regard to phonation, various methods have been proposed and used by many clinicians and researchers all over the world. Unfortunately, none of these methods appears to be standardized on an international basis. For some of these techniques, such as stroboscopy of the vibrating vocal folds, airflow measurement, measurement of the maximum phonation time and determination of the speech and vocal range, a majority of investigators seem to be in agreement in terms of the significance of these tests and the interpretation of the data thereby obtained. It might be a good time to discuss standardization of the clinical examination of voice.

In Japan, the Society of Logopedics and Phoniatrics set up a committee to study "Phonatory Function Tests" in 1975. The present author happened to be the chairman of this committee. The committee worked extensively until 1978 when some tentative conclusions were reached. Most of these conclusions are included in this book.

It would be the author's pleasure if this book could become one of the cornerstones for the standardization of the clinical examination of voice.

The author is greatly indebted to Dr. Barry D. Wyke for his tremendous thoughtfulness in correcting English.

Kurume, October 1981                                                    **M. Hirano**

# Contents

# Outline of Voice Production and Its Examination  1

Voice production involves a complex and precise control by the central nervous system of a series of events in the peripheral phonatory organs. Effective use of various methods of the clinical examination of the voice, applicable to each subject or patient, calls for a thorough understanding of the process of voice production and the significance and the nature of each clinical test. In this chapter, an outline of the process of voice production, including the clinical physiology and anatomy of the voice organs, is presented. Each clinical test item, then, is briefly explained and related to the process of voice production.

## A. Control of Voice Production

Although voice is occasionally produced involuntarily or reflexly, it is uttered, in most instances in human life, when man communicates via speech. Voice is also used in artistic activities including singing and theatrical performance. In other words, the human behavior associated with phonation is developed by learning. Thus, voice production is controlled by the brain.

Fig. 1.1 schematically represents the process of voice production and its control system. During speech and singing, the higher-order centers including the speech centers in the cerebral cortex first determine the sequence of sound production. The higher-order centers include the centers of linguistic and artistic activities. The command from the higher-order centers is transmitted to the motor cortex which is located in the precentral gyrus. The motor cortex gives a series of commands to the motor nuclei in the brain stem and the spinal cord which, in turn, transmit the commands to the respiratory, laryngeal and articulatory muscles. The extrapyramidal system which includes some parts of the cerebral cortex, the cerebellum and the

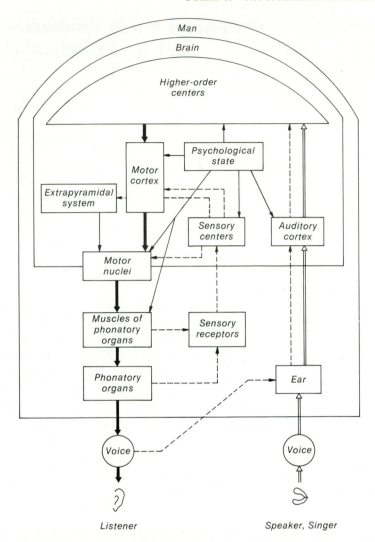

Fig. 1.1. A schematical presentation of the process of voice production and its control systems

basal ganglia, provides additional fine regulation of the activity of the respiratory, laryngeal and articulatory musculature.

The activity of these muscles results in movements of the phonatory organs, which produce a series of sounds known as voice. It is transmitted to the listener's ear.

The voice is also transmitted to the speaker's or singer's ear and is checked against the sound as has been preplanned (feed-back). Feed-back mechanisms also operate via the deep and superficial sensory receptors which provide information about the muscular contraction and the movements of the phonatory organs.

Psychological states can affect any aspect of the entire sequence of phonation. The autonomic nervous system may be involved.

# B. The Peripheral Process of Voice Production

All the activity in the central nervous system is finally reflected in muscular activity of the voice organ. In the majority of cases, parameters in the peripheral process of voice production are measured or evaluated during clinical examination of voice. Table 1.1 outlines the peripheral processes involved in the production and perception of voice, and the parameters to be determined or estimated at each level during the entire process of voice production.

Table 1.1. *Parameters in the peripheral process of the production and perception of voice (Hirano, 1975, modified)*

| | Parameters which regulate vibratory pattern of vocal fold | | Parameters which specify vibratory pattern | Parameters which specify sound generated | |
|---|---|---|---|---|---|
| Level | Physiological | Physical | Physical | Acoustic | Psycho-acoustic |
| Parameters | Neuromuscular control<br>Respiratory muscles<br>Laryngeal muscles<br><br><br><br><br>Articulatory muscles | (Primary)<br><br>Expiratory force<br>Vocal fold<br>  Position<br>  Shape & size<br>  Elasticity<br>  Viscosity<br>State of vocal tract<br>(Secondary)<br>Pressure drop across glottis<br>Volume velocity<br>Glottal impedance | Fundamental period<br>Symmetry<br>Periodicity<br>Uniformity<br>Glottal closure<br>Amplitude<br>Mucosal wave<br>Speed of excursion<br>Glottal area wave form | Fundamental frequency<br>Amplitude (Intensity)<br>Wave form<br>Acoustic spectrum<br>Fluctuation | Pitch<br><br>Loudness<br><br>Quality<br><br>Fluctuation |

The crucial event essential for voice production is vibration of the vocal folds. It changes DC air stream to AC air stream, converting aerodynamic energy to acoustical energy. From this point of view, the parameters involved in the process of phonation can be divided into three major groups:

(1) The parameters which regulate the vibratory pattern of the vocal folds.
(2) The parameters which specify the vibratory pattern of the vocal folds.
(3) The parameters which specify the nature of the sound generated.

The parameters which regulate the vibratory pattern of the vocal folds can be divided into two groups: physiological and physical. The physiological factors are, succinctly put, related to the activity of the respiratory, phonatory and articulatory muscles. The physical factors include the expiratory force, the condition of the vocal folds, and the state of the vocal tract. The expiratory force is the energy source of phonation and is regulated chiefly by the respiratory muscles and the state of the bronchopulmonary system and of the thoracic cage. The condition of the vocal

1 *

folds, which are the vibrators, is described with respect to the position, shape, size, elasticity and viscosity of the vocal folds. It is influenced by the activity of the laryngeal muscles, and pathological conditions of the vocal folds and the adjacent structures. The state of the vocal tract, the channel between the glottis and the lips, affects the vibratory pattern of the vocal folds to a certain extent and it is regulated chiefly by the articulatory muscles.

These primary physical factors in turn determine certain secondary features, which include the pressure drop across the glottis, volume velocity or mean airflow rate, and glottal impedance or mean glottal resistance. These secondary features are referred to as the aerodynamic parameters.

The vibratory pattern of the vocal folds can be described with respect to various parameters including the fundamental period or fundamental frequency, regularity or periodicity in successive vibrations, symmetry between the two vocal folds, uniformity or homogeneity in the movement of different points within each vocal fold, glottal closure during vibration, amplitude of vibration, speed of excursion, wave which travels on the mucosa, contact area between the two vocal folds, glottal area wave form, and so on.

The nature of the sound generated is determined chiefly by the vibratory pattern of the vocal folds. It can be specified both in acoustic terms and in psycho-acoustic terms. The psycho-acoustic parameters are naturally dependent on the acoustic parameters. The acoustic parameters are fundamental frequency, intensity, wave form or acoustic spectrum, and their time-related variations. The psycho-acoustic parameters are pitch, loudness and quality of the voice and their time-related variations.

# C. The Structure and Control of the Vocal Fold as a Vibrator

The vocal fold has a unique structure and is intricately controlled by the activity of the laryngeal muscles. In contrast to musical instruments which have multiple strings, humans use only a single pair of vocal folds to produce great varieties of fundamental frequencies, intensities and tonal qualities of voice. The secret of this phenomenon lies in the structure and the control of the human vocal fold. Derangements of the normal structure and the control of the vocal fold result in voice disorders.

## 1. Structure of the Vocal Fold as a Vibrator

The vocal fold has a layered-structure.

Fig. 1.2 shows a frontal section through the middle of the membraneous portion of a human vocal fold. It is the area at and around the edge of this part of the membraneous portion of the vocal fold that moves most markedly during phonation. From a histological point of view, one can differentiate the following five layers:

(1) The epithelium, which is of the squamous cell type. It can be regarded as a thin and stiff capsule whose purpose is to maintain the shape of the vocal fold;

(2) The superficial layer of the lamina propria, which consists of loose fibrous components and matrix. It can be regarded as somewhat like a mass of soft gelatin;

(3) The intermediate layer of the lamina propria, which consists chiefly of elastic fibers and can be likened to a bundle of soft rubber bands;

(4) The deep layer of the lamina propria, which primarily consists of collagenous fibers and something like a bundle of cotton thread; and

(5) The vocalis muscle, which constitutes the main body of the vocal fold and is like a bundle of rather stiff rubber bands.

The superficial layer of the lamina propria is referred to as Reinke's space. The portion which consists of the intermediate and deep layers of the lamina propria is known as the vocal ligament. From a mechanical point of view, the five layers can be reclassified into three sections: the *cover*, consisting of the epithelium and the superficial layer of the lamina propria; the *transition*, consisting of the intermediate and deep layers of the lamina propria; and the *body*, which consists of the vocalis muscle.

This layered structure of the vocal folds is of great significance in three aspects. First, each layer has a different mechanical property. Second, the mechanical properties of the outer four layers that constitutes the mucous membrane are controlled passively, whereas the mechanical properties of the innermost layer are regulated

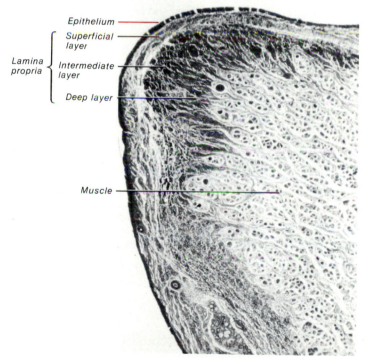

Fig. 1.2. A frontal section of a human vocal fold through the middle of the membraneous portion
(Hirano, 1977)

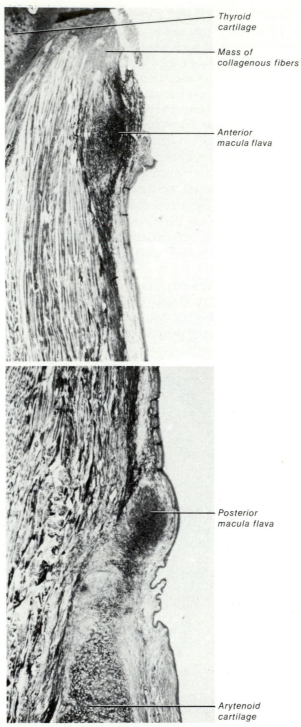

Fig. 1.3. Horizontal sections of a human vocal fold at the anterior and the posterior ends of the membraneous portion

both actively and passively. Third, almost all pathologies of the vocal folds originate from a specific layer.

The layered structure is not uniform along the length of the vocal fold (Fig. 1.3). At the anterior end of the vocal fold, there is a mass of collagenous fibers which appears to be connected to the inner perichondrium of the thyroid cartilage anteriorly and to the deep layer of the lamina propria posteriorly. Posterior to this mass of collagenous fibers, there is another mass of elastic fibers called the anterior macula flava. This is a continuation of the intermediate layer of the lamina propria. Similar variations are found near the posterior end of the membraneous part of the vocal fold. These masses of fibers near both ends of the vocal fold appear to act like cushions, which serve to protect the ends from the mechanical damage which may result during vibration of the vocal folds.

Towards the anterior and the posterior ends, the intermediate layer of the lamina propria becomes thicker, whereas the superficial layer, which is the most pliant among the layers, becomes thinner. Thus, the vocal fold appears to be the most pliable at the middle of its membraneous part, not only because of its location but also because of its structure.

## 2. Control of the Vocal Fold

*Function of the Laryngeal Muscles.* The laryngeal muscles are of great importance in regulating the mechanical properties of the vocal folds, that is, the vibrator. They control not only the position and shape of the vocal folds, but also the elasticity and viscosity of each layer of the vocal fold. Fig. 1.4 and Table 1.2 show the function of the five major intrinsic laryngeal muscles.

### (1) The Cricothyroid Muscle

The cricothyroid muscle brings the vocal folds to the line between the anterior commissure and the posterior cricoarytenoid ligament. In other words, when the cricothyroid muscle contracts the vocal folds are brought into a paramedian position. The level of the vocal fold within the larynx is lowered. The entire vocal fold is stretched, elongated and thinned. The edge of the vocal fold becomes sharp. All the layers are thereby passively stiffened.

Table 1.2. *Characteristic functions of the laryngeal muscles in vocal fold adjustments*

|  | CT | VOC | LCA | IA | PCA |
|---|---|---|---|---|---|
| Position | Paramed | *Adduct* | *Adduct* | *Adduct* | *Abduct* |
| Level | Lower | Lower | *Lower* | 0 | *Elevate* |
| Length | *Elongate* | *Shorten* | Elongate | (Shorten) | *Elongate* |
| Thickness | *Thin* | *Thicken* | Thin | (Thicken) | Thin |
| Edge | *Sharpen* | *Round* | Sharpen | 0 | Round |
| Muscle (Body) | *Stiffen* | *Stiffen* | Stiffen | (Slacken) | Stiffen |
| Mucosa (Cover and Transition) | *Stiffen* | *Slacken* | Stiffen | (Slacken) | Stiffen |

0: no effect,   ( ): slightly,   Italics: markedly.
CT: the cricothyroid muscle, VOC: the vocalis muscle, LCA: the lateral cricoarytenoid muscle,
IA: the interarytenoid muscle, PCA: the posterior cricoarytenoid muscle

## (2) The Vocalis Muscle

The vocalis muscle adducts the vocal folds, especially at the membraneous portions. It lowers, shortens and thickens the vocal fold. The edge of the vocal fold is rounded by contraction of the vocalis muscle. When the vocalis muscle is activated, the mus-

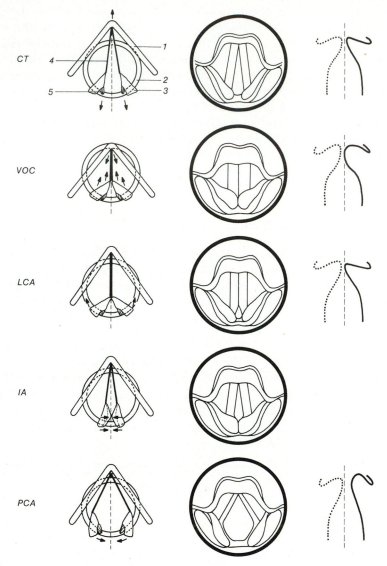

Fig. 1.4. A schematic presentation of the function of the laryngeal muscles. The left column shows the location of the cartilages and the edge of the vocal folds when the laryngeal muscles are activated individually. The arrow indicates the direction of the force exerted. *1* the thyroid cartilage, *2* the cricoid cartilage, *3* the arytenoid cartilage, *4* the vocal ligament, *5* the posterior cricoarytenoid ligament. The middle column shows views from above. The right column presents contours of frontal sections at the middle of the membraneous portion of the vocal fold. The dotted line shows a control where no muscle is activated

cular layer, which is the body of the vocal fold is actively stiffened, whereas the cover and transition layers are passively slackened.

### (3) The Lateral Cricoarytenoid Muscle

The lateral cricoarytenoid muscle adducts and lowers the tip of the vocal process of the arytenoid cartilage, and thus, adducts and lowers the entire vocal fold. When the lateral cricoarytenoid muscle is activated, the vocal fold is elongated and thinned. The edge of the vocal fold becomes sharp. All the layers are passively stiffened.

### (4) The Interarytenoid Muscle

The interarytenoid muscle adducts the vocal fold chiefly at the cartilaginous portion. It controls the position of the vocal fold, but does not affect the mechanical property of the vocal fold significantly.

### (5) The Posterior Cricoarytenoid Muscle

The posterior cricoarytenoid muscle abducts and elevates the tip of the vocal process of the arytenoid cartilage. Therefore, it abducts and elevates the entire vocal fold. When the posterior cricoarytenoid muscle is activated, the vocal fold is markedly elongated. The vocal fold becomes thin. The edge of the vocal fold is rounded. All the layers of the vocal fold are passively stiffened.

During actual phonation, the vocal fold is controlled by combined activity of the muscles discussed above.

## D. Outline of Clinical Examination of Voice

Diagnostic procedures for voice disorder comprise tests that elicit information regarding the actual process of voice production and the nature of the sound generated. The purposes of the diagnostic procedures are:
    (1) To determine the cause of a voice disorder,
    (2) To determine the degree and extent of the causative disease,
    (3) To evaluate the degree of disturbance in phonatory function,
    (4) To determine the prognosis of the voice disorder as well as that of the cause of the disorder, and
    (5) To establish a therapeutic programme.

Table 1.3 demonstrates the ways of direct or indirect assessment, observation and/or measurement of the parameters involved in the process of voice production. Many of such diagnostic modalities are not specific to voice disorders.

In this book, only selected clinical examinations which are specific or directly related to voice will be described. Electromyography is a test which evaluates some of the parameters which regulate the vibratory pattern of the vocal folds at the physiological level. Aerodynamic measurements deal with the aerodynamic factors. Procedures including stroboscopy, ultra high speed cinematography and glottography are used to examine the vibratory pattern of the vocal folds. Acoustic

Table 1.3. *Ways of direct or indirect assessment, observation and/or measurement of the parameters in the process of the production and perception of voice (Hirano, 1975, modified)*

| | Parameters which regulate vibratory pattern of vocal fold | | Parameters which specify vibratory pattern | Parameters which specify sound generated | |
|---|---|---|---|---|---|
| Level | Physiological | Physical | Physical | Acoustic | Psycho-acoustic |
| Ways of direct or indirect assessment, observation and/or measurement | History-taking<br>Physical examinations<br>Neurological examinations<br>Function tests<br>Endoscopy<br>X-ray examinations<br>Electromyography<br>Aerodynamic measurements<br>Histological examinations<br>Microbiological examinations<br>Blood and serum examinations<br>Endocrinological examinations<br>Observations during surgery<br>Behavioral tests<br>Psychological examinations | | Stroboscopy<br>Ultra high speed cinematography<br>Glottography<br>  Photoelectric<br>  Electrical<br>  Ultrasonic | Acoustic analysis | Auscultation of voice<br>Psychological assessments |

analysis of the voice quantifies the parameters which determine the acoustic characteristics of the sound generated. Ausculation and psychological assessment of the voice deal with the parameters which relate to the sound at the psycho-acoustic level. There are some other tests which evaluate certain abilities of phonation, such as the duration a subject can sustain a note, the range of fundamental frequency or intensity of voice a subject can cover, how effectively the glottis converts the aerodynamic energy into acoustic energy (glottal efficiency), and so on.

In the following chapters, details of these selected clinical examinations will be described. However, it should be emphasized that any voice clinician, including otolaryngologists, phoniatricians, speech pathologists, and logopedists, should keep all the possible diagnostic procedures in mind, and should be ready to make use of them whenever necessary.

# References

Hirano, M. (1975): Phonosurgery. Basic and clinical investigations. Otologia (Fukuoka) *21*, 239—442.

Hirano, M. (1977): Structure and Vibratory Behavior of the Vocal Folds. In: Dynamic Aspects of Speech Production (Sawashima, M., Cooper, F. S., eds.), pp. 13—27. Tokyo: University of Tokyo Press.

Hirano, M. (1979): Physical and anatomical studies of the structure of the vocal folds in normal and pathological states. (NIH Conference on the Assessment of Vocal Pathology.)

Koike, Y., Hirano, M., Morio, M. (1976): Function of the laryngeal muscles on position and shape of the vocal cord. (Proceedings 16th International Congress of Logopedics and Phoniatrics.) Basel: Karger.

# Electromyography of Laryngeal Muscles   2

Electromyography is the only procedure that directly demonstrates muscular activity. Electromyography of the laryngeal muscles appears to have been routinely used in a fairly large number of clinics in Japan and European countries. It is very useful particularly as one of the methods of the clinical examination of vocal fold paralysis. It can be also effectively used in examining patients with functional voice disorders.

## 1. Nature of Muscle Action Potential

A muscle fiber maintains a steady potential across its membrane (inside negative) at rest. When a nerve impulse arrives at the nerve ending, a chemical transmitter substance, acetylcholine, is liberated from the nerve ending on to the motor end-plate of the muscle. This induces depolarization of the muscle fiber membrane, producing an action potential. The action potential is transmitted along the muscle fiber in both directions at a speed of approximately 4 meters per second, exciting the contractile mechanism of the fiber in its wake. The muscle fiber begins to contract after an interval of approximately 1 msec.

When an electrode is placed outside the muscle fiber membrane, the action potential can be recorded. Since the action potential is very small (in the order of 0.1 to 1 mV), an amplification is required in order to record it. The graphic display obtained in this way from several muscle fibers is called an electromyogram. The procedure to obtain an electromyogram is called electromyography and the apparatus for electromyographic recording is called an electromyograph. No action potential is recorded in a normal resting muscle.

A muscle consists of a number of muscle fibers which are organized into functional units, called, motor units. Each motor unit consists of a single nerve cell, called a lower motor neuron, and the muscle fibers which are innervated by its branches. A motor neuron has a cell body, several short processes called the dendrites, and a long process called the axon.

The number of the muscle fibers innervated by a single motor neuron differs from muscle to muscle. This number is referred to as the size of the motor unit, and its reciprocal is the innervation ratio.

During voluntary contraction of a normal muscle, all the muscle fibers innervated by a single lower motor neuron act together. The tiny action potentials of the muscle fibers are summed up and they produce a larger action potential. The potential produced by (and recorded from) a single motor unit is called a "single motor unit potential".

Under normal conditions, each motor unit is activated at random intervals and different motor units are activated asynchronously. During a weak voluntary contraction a small number of motor units are active. In the vicinity of the recording needle or the wire electrode, only a single unit may be active. Increases in the force of contraction are brought about by three mechanisms.

(1) Increase in number of motor units activated (recruitment).

(2) Increase in the frequency of impulses in each motor unit.

(3) Synchronization of different motor units. This occurs only in extremely strong contractions or in fatigue as far as normal muscle is concerned.

During a strong contraction, the frequently recurring action potentials of many motor units are so numerous that one cannot be distinguished from the other. The resulting record is called an "interference pattern".

## 2. Apparatus and Electrodes

The electromyograph essentially consists of an electrode system, an amplifier, a cathode-ray oscilloscope, a loudspeaker and a recording system.

Either of two types of electrode is used: a needle electrode or a hooked-wire electrode. In examining disorders of the motor units, a needle electrode should be used. In order to avoid interfering signals from adjacent muscles, a bipolar needle electrode is preferable to a monopolar concentric needle electrode (Dedo and Hall, 1969; Dedo, 1970). Recordings made from different points within a muscle are useful, because different motor unit patterns can be found in a given muscle.

When the kinesiological pattern of a muscle or that of a set of muscles is examined, hooked-wire electrodes should be used. Hooked-wire electrodes were first used for electromyography of the laryngeal muscle by Hirano and Ohala (1967, 1969). They have the following important advantages: (1) they offer mini-

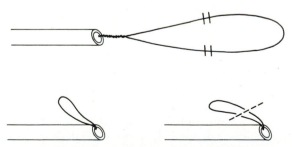

Fig. 2.1. The method of preparing a bipolar hooked-wire electrode (Hirano and Ohala, 1967, 1969)

mum discomfort to the subject, and consequently do not interfere with normal phonation; (2) they stay fairly well in place regardless of rapid movements of the vocal folds or the displacements of the entire larynx during phonation; and (3) they permit considerable localization of the area from which electrical activity is recorded.

Hirano and Ohala used a 40 gauge copper wire, 0.087 mm in diameter. Their method of electrode preparation is similar to that described by Basmajian and Stecko (1962) (Fig. 2.1). A single length of wire long enough to serve as two electrodes (50—60 cm) is cut. The free ends of the wire are twisted together and inserted into the bevelled end of a hypodermic needle. The wire is pulled through the needle until a small loop remains. The loop is bent back and cut leaving two ends (approximately 1 mm and 1.5 mm in length) protruding from the bevelled tip of the needle. At the other end of the wires the insulation is removed from the wires and these are connected to an amplifier.

Hirose (1971) adopted a platinum-iridium alloy wire with polyester coating, the diameter of which was approximately 0.05 mm. This wire is less easily bent than copper wire and is less springy than stainless steel. He also developed a probe which consists of an L-shaped metal rod and the shaft of a hypodermic needle (26 gauge), epoxybonded to the end of the shorter arm of the rod (Fig. 2.4).

# 3. Insertion of the Electrode into the Intrinsic Laryngeal Muscles

Faaborg-Andersen (1957), in his pioneering work on the electromyography of the laryngeal muscles, inserted a needle electrode into most of the intrinsic laryngeal muscle through the mouth. However, he inserted the electrode into the crico-thyroid muscle through the cervical skin. The presence of the needle electrode in the mouth and throat often makes it difficult for the subject to phonate normally. This technique, therefore, did not become popular in clinical examination.

Hiroto et al. (1962) described techniques of inserting needle electrodes into all the major intrinsic laryngeal muscles through the cervical skin. Their technique made it possible to use electromyography as a routine clinical procedure.

Hirano and Ohala (1967, 1969) developed a technique of placing hooked-wire electrodes into the major intrinsic laryngeal muscles through the cervical skin (Fig. 2.2). Their methods of insertion are essentially the same as those of Hiroto et al. The method of insertion into each muscle is as follows.

## The Cricothyroid Muscle

The skin is pierced at a point above the lower edge of the cricoid cartilage and lateral to the midline. The needle is directed posterolaterally and upwards aiming at the lower surface of the thyroid cartilage. If the electrodes are introduced beyond the inner surface of the thyroid cartilage, they may be placed in the lateral crico-arytenoid muscle instead. On the other hand, if the penetration is not deep enough, one may record activity from the sternohyoid muscle.

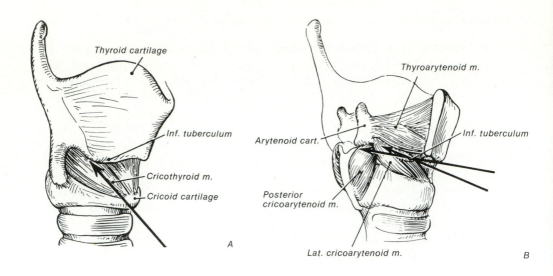

*Thyroid cartilage*

*Inf. tuberculum*

*Cricothyroid m.*

*Cricoid cartilage*

A

*Thyroarytenoid m.*

*Arytenoid cart.*

*Inf. tuberculum*

*Posterior cricoarytenoid m.*

*Lat. cricoarytenoid m.*

B

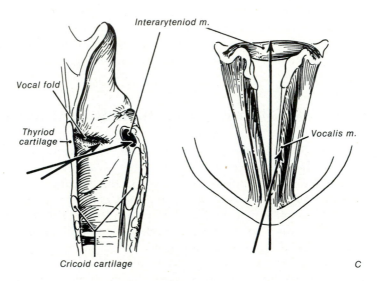

*Interaryteniod m.*

*Vocal fold*

*Thyriod cartilage*

*Vocalis m.*

*Cricoid cartilage*

C

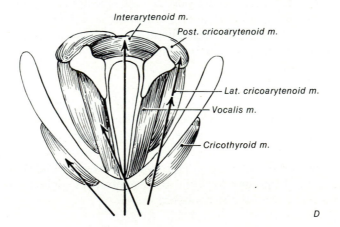

*Interarytenoid m.*

*Post. cricoarytenoid m.*

*Lat. cricoarytenoid m.*

*Vocalis m.*

*Cricothyroid m.*

D

## The Lateral Cricoarytenoid Muscle

The needle is inserted through the cricothyroid space penetrating the cricothyroid muscle anterior to the inferior tuberculum of the thyroid cartilage. The needle is directed posteriorly, laterally, and upwards, until the lateral cricoarytenoid muscle is pierced. If the needle is directed medially or too far upwards, it may be placed in the thyroarytenoid muscle.

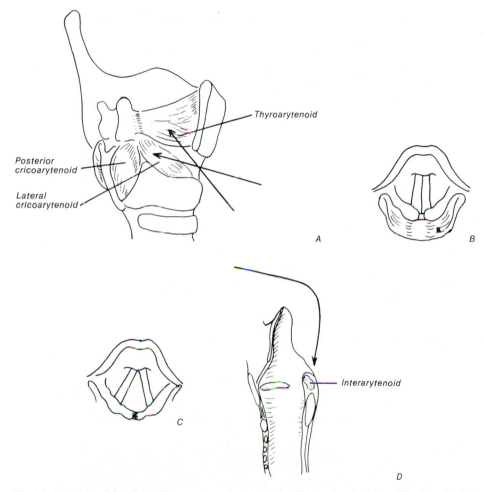

Fig. 2.3. Insertion of the electrode into the laryngeal muscles (Hirose, 1971). *A* A modified method of approaching the vocalis (thyroarytenoid) muscle. *B* Point of peroral insertion into the posterior cricoarytenoid muscle. *C* Point of peroral insertion into the interarytenoid muscle. *D* Peroral approach to the interarytenoid muscle

Fig. 2.2. Insertion of the electrodes into the laryngeal muscles (Hirano and Ohala, 1967, 1969): *A* The cricothyroid muscle. *B* The lateral and posterior cricoarytenoid muscles. *C* The vocalis and interarytenoid muscles. *D* Schematical presentation of the ways of insertion into the five major laryngeal muscles

### The Posterior Cricoarytenoid Muscle

The procedure is similar to that described for the lateral cricoarytenoid muscle, but the needle is inserted some 5—10 mm deeper. A slight downward tilt of the tip of the needle is often required to avoid hitting the arytenoid cartilage. For subjects with a narrow cricothyroid space, a slightly curved needle is helpful.

### The Vocalis Muscle

After topical anesthesia of the laryngeal mucosa, the needle is inserted into the sub-glottic space through the cricothyroid space at the midline. Then the tip of the needle is directed upwards and laterally (towards the vocal fold to be investigated). The mucosa of the lower surface of the vocal fold is penetrated until the exposed tips of the electrodes are located in the vocalis muscle. It is easier to insert the needle into the vocal fold during phonation than during respiration. The location of the electrodes can be confirmed by inspection with a laryngeal mirror.

### The Interarytenoid Muscle

Following local anesthesia of the laryngeal mucosa, the needle is inserted into the subglottal cavity through the cricothyroid space at the midline. The needle is pushed upwards and backwards. After piercing the anterior wall of the interaryte-noid area, the needle is placed in the interarytenoid muscle. The location of the electrodes can be monitored with a laryngeal mirror.

Hirose (1971) modified the Hirano and Ohala technique of inserting the electrodes into the vocalis muscle (Fig. 2.3A). In his modification, the skin is pierced at a point close to the midline at the level of the cricothyroid space. The needle is then directed cranially and slightly laterally. This method appears advantageous to that of Hirano and Ohala because the needle does not pass through the subglottic space but through the submucous tissue.

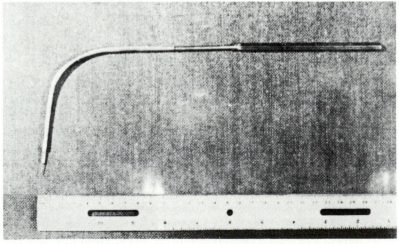

Fig. 2.4. The L-shaped probe used for peroral insertion (Hirose, 1971)

In the case of the posterior cricoarytenoid muscle, Hirose used the peroral insertion technique. It was for this purpose that he developed the L-shaped probe (Fig. 2.4). The insertion is performed under inspection with a laryngeal mirror. During insertion, the subject is placed in a sitting position and is asked to phonate a sustained vowel so as to open his hypopharyngeal lumen for easier access to the site of insertion, as illustrated in Fig. 3B. The electrodes are thus placed in the belly of the muscle on the cricoid cartilage through the hypopharyngeal mucosa. By this approach, there is little possibility of interference from neighboring muscles. This method is easier than that of Hirano and Ohala.

Hirose described a peroral approach for the interarytenoid muscle also. The same technique is used as described for the posterior cricoarytenoid and the insertion is made at the midline between the two arytenoid eminences (Fig. 3C, D).

## 4. Electromyographic Investigation of Vocal Fold Paralysis

Faaborg-Andersen (1957) investigated 27 patients with vocal fold paresis: 23 of whom had unilateral vocal fold paresis while the other 4 patients had bilateral paresis. Total denervation was not found in any of the patients, although 10 of the cases had resulted as a complication of thyroidectomy. In the majority of the single motor units investigated, the duration of action potential was longer in the paretic muscle than in the unaffected muscle, indicating a presence of a neurogenic paresis. The amplitude of the action potential of the paretic muscle was smaller than that of the normal side. Interference pattern was less marked on the paretic side, indicating loss of active motor units. Denervation potentials characterized by a short duration and a low amplitude were found in only one muscle. He reported that the crico-thyroid muscle presented abnormal activities in all the cases which had paretic vocal folds fixed in the intermediate position, and that it showed normal activities in all the cases whose paretic vocal folds were fixed in the paramedian or the median positions.

Sawashima *et al.* (1958) examined, using electromyography, 5 cases of recurrent laryngeal nerve paralysis. In 3 of the cases the paralysis was peripheral, and central in origin in the other 2 cases. No relationship was observed between the electro-myographic findings and the position of the paretic vocal fold. One of their cases, however, presented interesting findings. In this patient, bilateral paresis of the vocal folds had been caused by peri-esophagitis. The vocal folds were fixed in the intermediate position and all the laryngeal muscles except the cricothyroid showed electrical silence. A few months later, the patient recovered mobility of the vocal folds, but abduction was restricted. Electromyography revealed that the posterior cricoarytenoid was silent whereas the adductor muscles showed normal potentials. The authors also reported that normal electromyograms were obtained in two cases of ankylosis of the cricoarytenoid joint.

Šram *et al.* (1965) examined electromyographically patients with recurrent laryngeal nerve paralysis caused by thyroid surgery. They found, even in cases whose vocal folds clinically appeared totally paralyzed, some action potentials. They suggested that electromyography was useful in assessing the degree of such lesions and, therefore, helpful in determining the side to be subjected to lateral fixation of the vocal fold in cases of bilateral paralysis.

Using electromyography, Hirose *et al.* (1967) investigated 43 cases of recurrent laryngeal nerve palsy and related the results to the position of the paretic vocal fold. In 25 cases with the paretic vocal fold fixed in the median or in the paramedian positions, 21 showed action potentials in the vocalis muscle during voluntary action. In 18 cases with the paretic vocal fold fixed in the intermediate position, only 8 cases showed action potentials in the vocalis muscle associated with voluntary activity. Among these 8 cases, the cricothyroid muscle was electromyographically normal only in 2 cases and, in the remaining 6 cases, action potentials during phonation was reduced in the cricothyroid.

Tomita (1967) and Hiroto *et al.* (1968) reported their electromyographic findings in a total of 21 cases of unilateral vocal fold paralysis. They found four types of motor unit potentials in the muscles on the affected side: fibrillation voltages (fibrillation potentials), complex neuromuscular unit voltages (polyphasic potentials), reinnervation voltages (high amplitude potentials) and normal neuromuscular unit voltages (normal motor unit potentials). In all the cases, the interarytenoid muscle presented a normal electromyographic pattern. The cricothyroid muscle also presented a normal pattern except in one case. Eighteen of the 21 cases showed some potentials associated with voluntary activity, in either the thyroarytenoid, the lateral cricoarytenoid or posterior cricoarytenoid muscles, indicating an incomplete paralysis. Fibrillation potentials were present in some cases 22 days to 6 months after the onset of paralysis. Polyphasic potentials were recorded in cases 6 weeks to 6 months after the onset of the paralysis. High amplitude potentials were found only in 2 cases, one of which was 4 months and the other 57 months after the onset of the paralysis. Nine cases presented evidence of misdirected regenerating nerve fibers in one or more muscles. Two cases had restricted abduction of the paretic vocal fold; the vocal fold could move between the median position and the intermediate position, but could not be abducted beyond the intermediate position. In these two cases abnormal electromyograms were recorded mainly from the posterior cricoarytenoid muscle.

Ueda (1968a, b) reported results of a follow-up study on cases of postoperative recurrent laryngeal nerve paralysis. In 59 cases he repeated the electromyography at various intervals. The paralysis resulted after thyroid surgery in 56 cases and surgery for patent ductus arteriosus in 3 cases. Twenty-four cases recovered mobility of the vocal folds within 120 days after the surgery. Many of them presented electrical silence and/or low amplitude potentials between the 10th and the 20th postoperative days. After the 21st postoperative day, normal potentials appeared and their number increased in the course of time. These cases did not present fibrillation potentials or polyphasic potentials. This indicated that the lesion was not denervation but a neurapraxia or a temporary block. The remaining 35 cases did not recover mobility of the paretic vocal fold 1 to 2 years after the surgery. Most of these latter cases did not exhibit electrical potentials until about 30 days after surgery, when fibrillation potentials began to occur. Polyphasic potentials first appeared 50 days after the surgery in one case and were found in many cases after the 90th postoperative day. High amplitude potentials were found only in one case 110 days after surgery, and low amplitude potentials were first observed 90 days postoperatively. Normal potentials started occurring between the 80th and 120th postoperative days. After the 240th postoperative day many cases presented low amplitude and/ or normal potentials, but others showed no action potentials (electrical silence). The number of normal potentials observed was fewer than those observed in the normal muscles. The findings in the cases which failed to recover indicated that denervation had developed.

Dedo (1970) reported his electromyographic findings of 52 patients. Most of the patients who had paralyzed vocal fold(s) fixed in the paramedian position presented an electromyographic evidence of pure and total recurrent laryngeal nerve paralysis. Most of the patients with paralyzed vocal fold(s) fixed in the inter- mediate position showed electromyographic evidence of a paralysis of the recurrent and superior laryngeal nerves. Incomplete paralysis was observed only in 2 cases. In 4 patients electromyography revealed the presence of isolated superior laryngeal nerve paralysis. Their vocal folds were fully mobile but slightly bowed during phonation.

Table 2.1. *Electromyographic patterns in relation to the duration of vocal fold paralysis (Hirano et al., 1974)*

| Muscle | EMG | −2W | 2W−1M | 1M−2M | 2M−3M | 3M−6M | 6M−12M | 12M− | Total |
|---|---|---|---|---|---|---|---|---|---|
| VOC | S | 0 | 3 | 1 | 1 | 2 | 3 | 6 | 16 |
|  | F | 1 | 3 | 11 | 5 | 6 | 0 | 5 | 31 |
|  | P | 0 | 0 | 0 | 1 | 4 | 2 | 0 | 7 |
|  | H | 0 | 0 | 1 | 0 | 0 | 0 | 0 | 1 |
|  | N or n | 3 | 3 | 15 | 2 | 5 | 4 | 3 | 35 |
|  | Total | 4 | 9 | 28 | 9 | 17 | 9 | 14 | 90 |
| LCA | S | 1 | 2 | 0 | 0 | 3 | 2 | 3 | 11 |
|  | F | 1 | 6 | 7 | 7 | 8 | 0 | 4 | 33 |
|  | P | 0 | 0 | 0 | 3 | 6 | 5 | 1 | 15 |
|  | H | 0 | 0 | 1 | 0 | 1 | 1 | 0 | 3 |
|  | N or n | 2 | 8 | 25 | 5 | 9 | 6 | 13 | 68 |
|  | Total | 4 | 16 | 33 | 15 | 27 | 14 | 21 | 130 |
| PCA | S | 0 | 2 | 0 | 0 | 3 | 2 | 6 | 13 |
|  | F | 0 | 5 | 11 | 7 | 4 | 0 | 4 | 31 |
|  | P | 0 | 0 | 0 | 1 | 0 | 3 | 0 | 4 |
|  | H | 0 | 0 | 1 | 0 | 0 | 0 | 0 | 1 |
|  | N or n | 2 | 3 | 14 | 4 | 5 | 7 | 9 | 44 |
|  | Total | 2 | 10 | 26 | 12 | 12 | 12 | 19 | 93 |

S: Electrical silence, F: Fibrillation potential, P: Polyphasic potential, H: High amplitude potential, n: Normal potential (reduced in number), N: Normal potential.

When two or more different patterns were observed within a given muscle, the categorization in this table was made according to the following rule: F + S → F, P + x → P (x: any pattern), H + x → H, n + S and/or F → n, N + S and/or F → N.

Fex and Elmqvist (1973) conducted electromyographic investigations in 12 patients who had developed recurrent laryngeal nerve paresis following Hong-Kong-flu. Four patients had bilateral paresis whilst 8 had unilateral paresis. About 10 months after the occurrence of the paresis, good reinnervation was demonstrable in 12 of the still paretic vocal folds. Good or excellent glottic waves (wave running on the mucosa) during vocal fold vibration were also observed under stroboscopic light in these cases.

Hirano *et al.* (1974) investigated 130 cases of unilateral recurrent laryngeal nerve paralysis electromyographically. The vocalis muscle was investigated in 90, the lateral cricoarytenoid in 130, the posterior cricoarytenoid in 93, and the crico-thyroid in 116 cases. The cricothyroid muscle presented an abnormal pattern in only 10 cases. The discussion was, therefore, centered mainly on the vocalis, lateral cricoarytenoid and posterior cricoarytenoid muscles. Six different electromyo-graphic patterns were observed: electrical silence (S), fibrillation potentials (F), polyphasic potentials (P), high amplitude potentials (H), normal potentials but reduced in number (n), and normal potentials which were almost normal in number (N). Tables 2.1 and 2.2 show their results.

Table 2.2. *Electromyographic patterns where the findings in three muscles of each case were put together. The same rule for categorization as that in Table 2.1 was applied (Hirano et al., 1974)*

| | |
|---|---:|
| Silent | 8 |
| Fibrillation | 31 |
| Polyphasic | 14 |
| High amplitude | 3 |
| Normal (Reduction in active units) | 49 |
| Normal (Marked misdirected reinnervation in 10) | 25 |
| Total | 130 |

The authors discussed the relation between the electromyographic patterns and the duration of paralysis, differences in the vulnerability and recovery of the muscles, the relation between the electromyographic findings and the position of the paretic vocal fold, the relation between the electromyographic findings and the cause of paralysis, and prognostic significance of the electromyographic findings. The results can be summarized as follows: (1) In 91 of 130 cases, some action poten-tials associated with voluntary movement were found; thus they showed incom-plete paralysis where the motor units were partially innervated. (2) Fibrillation potentials were found at the earliest 12 days after the onset of paralysis. Polyphasic potentials were present at the earliest 2 months after the onset. (3) No difference in vulnerability or in recovery was observed to exist between the different muscles in most clinical cases. (4) All the 20 cases which had restricted mobility of the paretic vocal fold showed action potentials associated with voluntary movement. (5) In 110 cases with fixed vocal folds, no significant relationship between the electromyo-graphic findings and the position of the paretic vocal folds were observed. Abnor-mality in the cricothyroid muscle bore no significant relationship to the position of the paretic fold. (6) Action potentials induced by voluntary activity were observed to a significant extent in cases where the cause of the paralysis was a cold or unknown. (7) From a prognostic point of view, the most important finding in these electromyographic investigations was the presence of action potentials associated with voluntary activity.

Hirano (1975) and Hirano *et al.* (1977) reported their results of investigations in which a total of 52 cases of recurrent laryngeal nerve paralysis of varied etiologies were followed for a year or more, in which they had related their electromyographic findings to the prognosis. The most important factor, for prognostic purposes, was the presence of action potentials induced by voluntary activity. Ten cases were subjected to electromyography within a month after the onset of paralysis. Five of them showed voluntary action potentials whereas the other 5 did not. Electromyography was not significant in determining prognosis during this period. In 14 other cases examined electromyographically 1 to 3 months after the onset, 8 cases showed voluntary action potentials and 6 cases did not. Five of the former recovered mobility later to different degrees, whereas none in the latter group improved. Three to 6 months after the onset of paralysis, electromyography was performed on 14 other cases. Eleven cases demonstrated voluntary action potentials, with the paretic vocal fold fixed in the median position in 6 cases and in the paramedian position in the other 5 cases. Five of the former recovered mobility while none of the latter recovered. No voluntary action potentials were observed in the remaining 3 cases, and only 1 in this group recovered mobility to some extent. Lastly, in the 14 cases examined 6 months or more after the onset, 6 cases showed voluntary action potentials and 8 cases did not. None of these 14 cases recovered mobility.

In summary, the significance of electromyography for vocal fold paralysis seems to be as follows:

(1) Electromyography is helpful in differentiating vocal fold paralysis from immobility of the vocal folds caused by various mechanical fixations.

(2) Electromyography gives information about the degree and the extent of paralysis.

(3) It is useful in determining the side to subject to lateral fixation of the vocal fold in cases of bilateral vocal fold paralysis.

(4) It is helpful from a prognostic point of view. The presence of action potentials induced by voluntary activity indicates a favorable prognosis.

## 5. Electromyography of Functional Voice Disorders

Šram and Kalvodová (1965) reported their electromyographic findings in patients with psychogenic aphonia and in those with spastic dysphonia. The vocalis muscles showed irregular activities during normal and deep breathing. In psychogenic aphonia, there was no consistent picture of the pattern and duration of interference potentials during attempted phonation: the potentials either decreased, disappeared or temporarily increased. In spastic dysphonia, an increase in tension of the vocalis muscle was found at rest as well as during phonation.

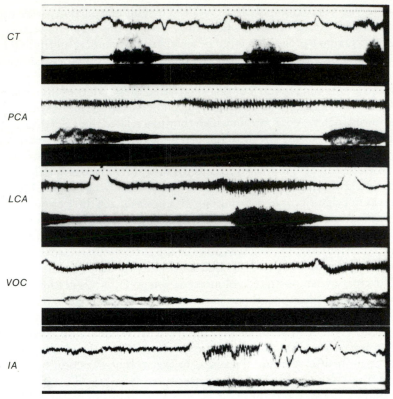

Fig. 2.5. Electromyograms of the laryngeal muscles of a patient with psychogenic dysphonia

Fig. 2.5 shows the electromyograms of a patient with psychogenic dysphonia who was treated at Kurume University Hospital. Her larynx appeared normal during respiration under observation with a laryngeal mirror. When she attempted to phonate the posterior part of the glottis was not completely closed. Electromyography revealed that the posterior cricoarytenoid was active during phonation as well as during inspiration. The cricothyroid and the adductor muscles showed normal patterns of activity. The incomplete glottic closure during phonation could be attributed to the neutralization of the activity of the adductor muscles as a result of the contraction of the posterior cricoarytenoid muscle.

# References

Atkins, J. P., jr. (1973): An electromyographic study of recurrent laryngeal nerve conduction and its clinical applications. Laryngoscope *83*, 796–807.

Basmajian, J. V., Stecko, G. (1962): A new bipolar electrode for electromyography. J. Appl. Physiol. *17*, 849.

Brewer, D. W., Briess, F. B., Faaborg-Andersen, K. (1960): Clinical testing versus electromyography. Ann. Otol. *69*, 781–804.

Dedo, H. (1970): The paralyzed larynx: An electromyographic study in dogs and humans. Laryngoscope *80*, 1455—1517.

Dedo, H. H., Hall, W. N. (1969): Electrodes in laryngeal electromyography. Reliability comparison. Ann. Otol. *78*, 172—180.

Faaborg-Andersen, K. (1957): Electromyographic investigation of intrinsic laryngeal muscles in humans. Acta Physiol. Scand. *41*, Suppl. 140, 9—148.

Fex, S. (1970): Judging the movements of vocal cords in larynx paralysis. Acta Otolaryngol. *263*, 82—83.

Fex, S., Elmqvist, D. (1973): Endemic recurrent laryngeal nerve paresis. Correlation between EMG and stroboscopic findings. Acta Otolaryngol. *75*, 368—369.

Fex, S., Henriksson, B. (1970): Phoniatric treatment combined with radiotherapy of laryngeal cancer for the avoidance of radiation damage. Acta Otolaryngol. *263*, 128—129.

Haglund, S. (1973): The normal electromyogram in human cricothyroid. Acta Otolaryngol. *75*, 448 to 453.

Hirano, M. (1975): Phonosurgery. Basic and clinical investigations. Otologia (Fukuoka) *21*, 239—440.

Hirano, M. (1976): Clinical examination for voice disorders in recurrent laryngeal nerve palsy. XVIth Int. Congr. Logopedics and Phoniatrics, 159—167.

Hirano, M., Koike, Y., Joyner, J. (1969): Style of phonation. An electromyographic investigation of some laryngeal muscles. Arch. Otolaryngol. *89*, 902—908.

Hirano, M., Nozoe, I., Shin, T., Maeyama, T. (1974): Electromyographic findings in recurrent laryngeal nerve paralysis. A study of 130 cases. Pract. Otol. Kyoto *67*, 231—242.

Hirano, M., Ohala, J. (1967): Use of hooked-wire electrodes for electromyography of the intrinsic laryngeal muscles. Working Papers in Phonetics UCLA *7*, 35—45.

Hirano, M., Ohala, J. (1969): Use of hooked-wire electrodes for electromyography of the intrinsic laryngeal muscles. J. Sp. Hear. Res. *12*, 362—373.

Hirano, M., Ohala, J., Smith, T. (1967): Current techniques in obtaining EMG data. Working Paper in Phonetics UCLA *7*, 20—24.

Hirano, M., Ohala, J., Vernnard, W. (1969): The function of laryngeal muscles in regulating fundamental frequency and intensity of phonation. J. Sp. Hear. Res. *12*, 616—628.

Hirano, M., Shin, T., Nozoe, I. (1977): Prognostic aspect of recurrent laryngeal nerve paralysis. IALP Congress Proceedings, 95—103.

Hirano, M., Vernnard, W., Ohala, J. (1970): Regulation of register, pitch and intensity of voice. An electromyographic investigation of intrinsic laryngeal muscles. Folia Phoniat. *22*, 1—20.

Hirose, H. (1971): Electromyography of the articulatory muscles: Current instrumentation and technique. Status Report on Speech Research (Haskins Lab.) *25/26*, 73—86.

Hirose, H., Gay, T. (1972): The activity of the intrinsic laryngeal muscles in voicing control: electromyographic study. Phonetica *25*, 140—164.

Hirose, H., Kobayashi, T., Okamura, M., Kurauchi, Y., Iwamura, S., Ushijuma, T., Sawashima, M. (1967): Recurrent laryngeal nerve palsy. J. Otolaryngol. Jpn. *70*, 1—17.

Hiroto, I., Hirano, M., Tomita, H. (1968): Electromyographic investigation of human vocal cord paralysis. Ann. Otol. *77*, 296—304.

Hiroto, I., Hirano, M., Toyozumi, Y., Shin, T. (1962): A new method of placement of a needle electrode in the intrinsic laryngeal muscles for electromyography. Insertion through the skin. Pract. Otol. (Kyoto) *55*, 499—504.

Hiroto, I., Hirano, M., Toyozumi, Y., Shin, T. (1967): Electromyographic investigation of the intrinsic laryngeal muscles related to speech sounds. Ann. Otol. *76*, 861—873.

Knutsson, E., Martensson, A., Martensson, B. (1969): The normal electromyogram in human vocal muscles. Acta Otolaryngol. *68*, 526—536.

Kotby, N. M. (1975): Percutaneous laryngeal electromyography standardization of the technique. Folia Phoniat. *27*, 116—127.

Luchsinger, R., Arnold, G. E. (1970): Handbuch der Stimm- und Sprachheilkunde. Wien-New York: Springer.

Satoh, I. (1978): Evoked electromyographic test applied for recurrent laryngeal nerve paralysis. Laryngoscope *88*, 2022—2031.

Sawashima, M., Sato, M., Funasaka, S., Totsuk, G. (1958): Electromyographic study of the human larynx and its clinical application. J. Otolaryngol. Jpn. *61*, 1357—1364.

Šram, F., Kalvodová, E. (1965): Elektromyographische Befunde bei psychogenen Aphonien und spa-
    stischen Dysphonien, Vol. II. Acta Soc., XII int. Logopead. et Phoniatr. Congress. Cited by Luch-
    singer and Arnold (1970).
Šram, F., Kalvodová, E., Drechsler, B. (1965): Elektromyographische Befunde bei Rekurrensparese und
    Strumektomie. Hals-Nas.-Ohr.-Tagung, Leipzig. Cited by Luchsinger and Arnold (1970).
Tomita, H. (1967): An electromyographic study of recurrent laryngeal nerve paralysis. J. Otolaryngol.
    Jpn. *70*, 963—985.
Ueda, N. (1968a): A clinical of the recurrent laryngeal nerve paralysis following surgical operations
    (Part I). Otologia (Fukuoka) *61*, 365—392.
Ueda, N. (1968b): Clinical investigations of postoperative recurrent laryngeal nerve paralysis (Part II).
    Hiroshima Medical J. *16*, 431—459.

# Aerodynamic Tests   **3**

## A. General Description

The aerodynamic aspect of phonation is characterized by four parameters: subglottal pressure, supraglottal pressure, glottal impedance and the volume velocity of the airflow at the glottis. The value of these parameters varies during one vibratory cycle according to the opening and closing of the glottis. These rapid variations in the values of the aerodynamic parameters cannot usually be measured in living humans because of technical difficulties.

For clinical purposes, the mean value of these parameters is usually determined. The four parameters are related as shown below:

$$P_{SUB} - P_{SUP} = MFR \times GR \tag{1}$$

where $P_{SUB}$ is the mean subglottal pressure; $P_{SUP}$, the mean supraglottal pressure; MFR, the mean flow rate represented as a unit of volume velocity; and GR, the mean glottal resistance. Strictly speaking, the "mean" used here implies the root mean square (rms) value.

When the phonation is associated with an open vocal tract, as in the case of open vowels, the supraglottal pressure is equal to the atmospheric pressure. In this circumstance, the following equation applies:

$$P_{SUB} = MFR \times GR \tag{2}$$

This relationship is analogous to the one which exists between voltage, current and resistance known as Ohm's law (Fig. 3.1).

The measurement of the mean flow rate is often done as an out-patient procedure. The determination of the subglottal pressure calls for an invasive approach. The glottal resistance cannot be directly measured, it is calculated from the mean flow rate and the mean subglottal pressure using Equation (2).

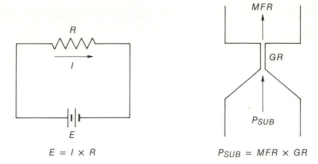

Fig. 3.1. Relationship between mean subglottal pressure *(P<sub>SUB</sub>)*, mean flow rate *(MFR)* and mean glottal resistance *(GR)* is analogous to that between the voltage *(E)*, current *(I)* and resistance *(R)*

# B. Airflow Rate

## 1. Apparatus for Airflow Measurement

### (1) Spirometer

Any kind of spirometer which is used to assess respiratory function can be utilized for airflow measurement during phonation. A spirometer is not an expensive apparatus and, is, therefore, available in many clinics.

    Major disadvantages of the spirometer are that other signals, such as acoustic signals, cannot be displayed simultaneously, and that the frequency response is poor. Nevertheless, the spirometer is used clinically to measure the mean airflow rate during sustained phonation. The use of the spirometer in the voice clinic was first proposed by Isshiki *et al.* (1967) and its usefulness has been confirmed by several investigators (Hirano, 1975; Shigemori, 1977; Yoshioka *et al.*, 1977).

### (2) Pneumotachograph

A pneumotachograph consists of three major components: a laminar air resistor, a differential pressure transducer, and an amplifying and recording system. When air flows through the resistor, a pressure difference is created across the resistor. Since the pressure difference is linearly related to the airflow rate under certain conditions, the airflow rate can be calculated by measuring the pressure difference. With the use of an integrating circuit, the airflow volume for a given time can be determined. When a polygraph system is used, some other signals related to phonation can be recorded simultaneously in addition to the airflow display. The frequency response of the pneumotachograph is not sensitive enough (usually flat for DC-50 Hz range) to register rapid variations of volume velocity.

    The pneumotachograph has been extensively used for clinical purposes (Isshiki and von Leden, 1964; Hirano *et al.*, 1968; Iwata and von Leden, 1970a).

*(3) Hot-Wire Anemometer*

The hot-wire anemometer is based on the principle that the heat removed from a hot-wire by a gas stream is linearly related to the square root of the velocity of the gas stream and that the voltage drop across the wire is linearly related to the square root of the the heat removed. Thus, the airflow velocity is calculated by measuring the electric voltage drop across the hot-wire. The old types of the hot-wire ane-mometer had such large time constants that they were not used for voice research. Recent advance in technology facilitated the development of a constant-tempera-ture type of hot-wire anemometer in which the temperature of the hot-wire is kept unchanged by supplying an appropriate electric current using a feedback circuitry. This type of hot-wire anemometer has a frequency response flat up to 1 KHz (Isshiki, 1977). Isshiki (1977), Saito (1977) and Kitajima *et al.* (1978) reported the advantages of this new type of hot-wire anemometer for clinical tests. One disad-vantage of the hot-wire anemometer is the fact that it cannot detect the direction of the air stream.

## 2. Measurement of the Mean Flow Rate

The mean flow rate of a sustained vowel (usually vowel /a/) has been used as a practical value for evaluating phonatory function. It is obtained by dividing the total volume of air used during phonation by the duration of phonation. During the clinical examination, the subject is requested to phonate at his/her natural pitch and loudness. Two manners of phonation have been adopted: maximum sustained phonation and phonation over a determined period.

The subject is instructed to phonate into a mask fitted tightly to the face, or into a mouth piece with the nose clamped. The mask or the mouth piece is coupled to a spirometer, a pneumotachograph or a hot-wire anemometer. Some pre-test practice is advisable to help the subject perform the task adequately.

## 3. Normal Values of the Mean Flow Rate

*(1) Habitual Phonation*

Normal values of the mean flow rate (MFR) of adults has been reported by several investigators (Table 3.1). The average values of the MFR range from 89 to 141 ml/sec. In Table 3.1, no consistent difference in MFR has been observed between the male and the female, either during maximum sustained phonation and the phonation over comfortable period, or between results obtained either with the spirometer or the pneumotachograph. In most reports, the value ranges approximately from 70 to 200 ml/sec. The critical region, which indicates the possible range for the normal population, is approximately from 40 to 200 ml/sec (Table 3.1). It appears reason-able to regard MFR values greater than 200 ml/sec or less than 40 ml/sec as abnor-mal, as far as phonation at a habitual pitch and loudness is concerned.

For normal children, Shigemori (1977) measured MFR in school children during phonation over a comfortable duration, with the use of a spirometer (Table

Table 3.1. *Normal values for mean flow rate (in ml/sec) in adults*

| Author(s) | | N | Average | Confidence limit | Critical region | Range | Apparatus used |
|---|---|---|---|---|---|---|---|
| Isshiki et al. (1967) | * | M 5<br>F 5 | 123.1<br>133.1 | | | 94.7–153.0<br>68.7–162.0 | Spirometer |
| Isshiki et al. (1967) | | M 5<br>F 5 | 126.2<br>135.9 | | | 104.7–164.3<br>69.0–171.0 | Pneumotachograph |
| Yanagihara et al. (1966) | * | M 11<br>F 11 | 112.0<br>100.0 | | | 70 –164<br>61 –130 | Pneumotachograph |
| Hirano et al. (1968) | * | M 25<br>F 25 | 101<br>92 | 86–117<br>79–107 | 46 –222<br>43 –197 | | Pneumotachograph |
| Yoshioka et al. (1977) | * | M 25<br>F 25 | 96<br>97 | | 44.9–147<br>13.0–181 | | Spirometer |
| Isshiki and von Leden (1964) | ** | M 36<br>F | 141<br>119 | 73–183 | | 109 –182<br>76 –172 | Pneumotachograph |
| Shigemori (1977) | ** | M 25<br>F 25 | 140<br>133 | 118–166<br>118–149 | 59 –336<br>73 –240 | 80 –305<br>85 –200 | Spirometer |
| Yoshioka et al. (1977) | ** | M 25<br>F 25 | 112<br>89 | | 66.5–162<br>37.6–140 | | Spirometer |

* During maximum sustained phonation.     ** During phonation over comfortable duration.

Table 3.2. *Normal values for mean flow rate (in ml/sec) in school children (Shigemori, 1977)*

| Grade Level | | Average | Confidence limit (95%) | Critical region (95%) | Range |
|---|---|---|---|---|---|
| 1st grade | male | 93 | 84—104 | 54—162 | 60—155 |
| | female | 95 | 84—109 | 49—185 | 55—175 |
| | total | 94 | 87—102 | 53—169 | 55—175 |
| 3rd grade | male | 119 | 106—133 | 66—212 | 65—185 |
| | female | 105 | 94—117 | 59—187 | 60—180 |
| | total | 111 | 103—121 | 63—197 | 60—185 |
| 5th grade | male | 110 | 97—124 | 59—202 | 70—200 |
| | female | 135 | 123—149 | 83—220 | 80—190 |
| | total | 119 | 110—130 | 65—218 | 70—200 |
| 7th grade | male | 147 | 132—163 | 85—253 | 80—210 |
| | female | 101 | 90—113 | 55—184 | 60—180 |
| | total | 122 | 111—134 | 62—239 | 60—210 |

3.2). She described that MFR was significantly smaller for the school children of the first grade than those of the other age groups. She also reported significant differences in MFR between boys and girls in the fifth and the seventh grades. Comparison of the values listed in Tables 3.1 and 3.2 leads to the conclusion that the normal standard for adults can also be applied to school children.

### (2) Variations in Vocal Intensity

Isshiki (1964, 1965b) reported that MFR tended to be more closely related to the intensity of voice at high pitch levels than at low pitch levels. Hirano *et al.* (1970) reported that the increase in MFR with increasing intensity was much greater in falsetto than in heavy, or modal, voice.

### (3) Variations in Vocal Register

Large *et al.* (1972) compared the MFR values of five male singers singing in the head register and in the falsetto voice at the same fundamental frequency and intensity. MFR was much greater in falsetto (ranging from 230 to 525 ml/sec, and an average of 398 ml/sec) than in the head register (ranging from 100 to 310 ml/sec, an average of 219 ml/sec). Hirano (1970) and Hirano *et al.* (1970) reported similar findings.

McGlone (1967) measured MFR in five male and five female subjects during vocal fry phonation and reported that the MFR ranged between 2.0 and 71.9 ml/sec. He did not find any consistent relationship between the MFR and the vocal fry frequency.

## 4. The Mean Flow Rate in Pathological States

### (1) Recurrent Laryngeal Nerve Paralysis

The MFR in cases of recurrent laryngeal nerve paralysis has been reported by several investigators (Table 3.3). In most cases, the MFR was greater than normal. There is a

Table 3.3. *Mean flow rate (in ml/sec) in recurrent laryngeal nerve paralysis*

| Author(s) | N | | Average | Range | Greater than critical region | Greater than 200 ml/sec | Greater than 300 ml/sec |
|---|---|---|---|---|---|---|---|
| Isshiki and von Leden (1964) | Intermediate | ? | 845 | 680–1150 | | | |
| | Paramed. Med. | ? | 346 | 192– 770 | | | |
| Hirano et al. (1968) | | 13 | | 53– 621 | 8 (62%) | | |
| Iwata et al. (1972) | Intermediate | 19 | 353 | | 15 (79%) | | |
| | Paramed. Med. | 16 | 249 | | 6 (38%) | | |
| | Bilateral | 7 | 234 | | 3 (43%) | | |
| Iwata et al. (1976) | Intermediate | 21 | 361 | 162– 692 | | | |
| | Paramedian | 16 | 248 | 71– 733 | | | |
| Shigemori (1977) | Unilateral | 113 | | 85– 957 | | 84 (74%) | 60 (53%) |
| | Bilateral | 9 | | 35– 590 | | 4 (44%) | 2 (22%) |
| Yoshioka et al. (1977) | Male | 14 | { 299 | | 12 (86%) | Maximum sustained phonation | |
| | | | { 328 | | 10 (71%) | Comfortable duration | |
| | Female | 14 | { 248 | | 8 (57%) | Maximum sustained phonation | |
| | | | { 222 | | 12 (71%) | Comfortable duration | |

tendency that the more laterally the paretic vocal fold is fixed the greater the MFR values. MFR is a good indicator of the phonatory function in recurrent laryngeal nerve paralysis and it can be used as a monitor of treatment (Hirano *et al.*, 1968; Hirano, 1975; Isshiki, 1977; Saito, 1977; Shigemori, 1977).

## *(2) Sulcus Vocalis*

According to Shigemori (1977), the MFR of 26 patients of sulcus vocalis ranged from 50 to 723 ml/sec. The MFR was greater than 200 ml/sec in 12 patients (46 per cent) and greater than 300 ml/sec in 6 patients (23 per cent).

## *(3) Laryngitis*

Table 3.4 presents the MFR in cases of laryngitis as measured by several investigators. In more than half the cases, the MFR lies within the normal range.

Table 3.4. *Mean flow rate (in ml/sec) during laryngitis*

| Author(s) | N | | Average | Range | Greater than critical region | Greater than 200 ml/sec | Greater than 300 ml/sec |
|---|---|---|---|---|---|---|---|
| Isshiki and von Leden (1964) | ? | | 173 | 53—440 | | | |
| Hirano *et al.* (1968) | 5 | | | 155—349 | 2 (40%) | | |
| Iwata *et al.* (1972) | M | 45 | 150 | | | | |
| | F | 23 | 137 | | | | |
| Iwata *et al.* (1976) | M | 64 | 166 | 65—500 | | | |
| | F | 32 | 146 | | | | |
| Shigemori (1977) | 59 | | | 35—559 | | 23 (39%) | 9 (15%) |

## *(4) The Nodule, Polyp and Polypoid Swelling of the Vocal Fold*

Table 3.5 presents MFR values in cases with nodule, polyp and polypoid swelling (Reinke's edema) of the vocal fold. In many cases, the value of the MFR exceeds the normal range, but not as marked as in cases with recurrent laryngeal nerve paralysis. Shigemori (1977) reported a positive relationship between the MFR and the size of the lesion. MFR is frequently decreased after surgical treatment of the lesion (Hirano, 1975; Saito, 1977; Shigemori, 1977).

## *(5) Tumor*

Table 3.6 shows the MFR values in cases with tumors of the vocal fold(s), most of which were neoplastic. The value of the MFR varied from patient to patient. Isshiki and von Leden reported that in the case of a large tumor, MFR always exceeded the normal range.

Table 3.5. *Mean flow rate (in ml/sec) associated with nodule, polyp and polypoid swelling of the vocal fold*

| Author(s) | N | | Average | Range | Greater than critical region | Greater than 200 ml/sec | Greater than 300 ml/sec |
|---|---|---|---|---|---|---|---|
| Hirano et al. (1968) | | 18 | | 39–379 | 5 (28%) | | |
| Iwata et al. (1972) | Nodule | 23 | 177 | | | | |
| | Polyp | 18 | 162 | | | | |
| Iwata et al. (1976) | Nodule | M 29 | 199 | 91–260 | | | |
| | | F 19 | 247 | | | | |
| | Polyp, unilat. | M 29 | 253 | 75–533 | | | |
| | | F 13 | 290 | | | | |
| | Polyp, bilat. | M 8 | 256 | 120–560 | | | |
| | | F 8 | 359 | | | | |
| | Polypoid | 6 | 437 | | | | |
| Shigemori (1977) | Nodule, Polyp | 182 | | 70–740 | | 103 (57%) | 45 (25%) |
| | Polypoid | 36 | | 75–697 | | 20 (55%) | 7 (19%) |
| Yoshioka et al. (1977) | | M 24 | 187 | | 15 (68%) | Maximum sustained phonation | |
| | | | 195 | | 14 (58%) | Comfortable duration | |
| | | F 19 | 174 | | 8 (42%) | Maximum sustained phonation | |
| | | | 171 | | 10 (53%) | Comfortable duration | |

Table 3.6. *Mean flow rate (in ml/sec) associated with vocal fold tumors*

| Author(s) | N | | Average | Range | Greater than critical region | Greater than 200 ml/sec | Greater than 300 ml/sec |
|---|---|---|---|---|---|---|---|
| Isshiki and von Leden (1964) | ? | Small tumor | 189 | 81–420 | | | |
| | ? | Large tumor | 259 | 189–385 | | | |
| Hirano et al. (1968) | 10 | Neoplasm | | 59–518 | 4 (40%) | | |
| Iwata et al. (1972) | 11 | Papilloma Fibroma } Leukoplakia | 227 | | 7 (64%) | | |
| | 13 | Malignant | 170 | | | | |
| Iwata et al. (1976) | 4 | Haemangioma | 191 | 73–274 | | | |
| | 12 | Papilloma | 319 | 42–346 | | | |
| | 26 | Carcinoma | 168 | 63–500 | | | |
| Shigemori (1977) | 28 | Benign mass | | 30–703 | | 15 (54%) | 6 (21%) |
| | 14 | Epithelial hyperplasia | | 33–220 | | 1 ( 7%) | 0 ( 0%) |
| | 34 | Carcinoma | | 75–350 | | 16 (47%) | 6 (18%) |

*(6) Contact Granuloma*

In cases with contact granuloma, MFR is usually within normal limits as shown in Table 3.7.

Table 3.7. *Mean flow rate (in ml/sec) associated with contact granuloma*

| Author(s) | N | Average | Range | Greater than critical region |
|---|---|---|---|---|
| Isshiki and von Leden (1964) | ? | 144 | 84–204 | |
| Hirano *et al.* (1968) | 5 | | 40–152 | 0 |
| Iwata *et al.* (1972) | 5 | 69 | | 0 |
| Iwata *et al.* (1976) | 5 | 68 | | |

*(7) Spastic Dysphonia*

Hirano *et al.* (1968) measured MFR in 8 cases with spastic dysphonia. The value ranged from 63 to 186 ml/sec and did not exceed the normal range in any case.

# C. Phonation Quotient

## 1. Definition

Phonation quotient (PQ) is defined as the value obtained when the vital cavity (VC) is divided by the maximum phonation time (MPT).

$$\text{Phonation quotient (PQ)} = \frac{\text{Vital capacity (VC)}}{\text{Maximum phonation time (MPT)}}$$

## 2. Relationship Between Phonation Quotient and Mean Flow Rate

The total air volume used during maximum sustained phonation (phonation volume, PV, by Yanagihara *et al.*, 1966) is usually less than the vital capacity (Gutzmann and Loewy, 1920; Yanagihara *et al.*, 1966; Yanagihara and Koike, 1967; Isshiki *et al.*, 1967; Yoshioka *et al.*, 1977). The ratio of PV to VC was found to be 50.4 to 73.0 per cent by Yanagihara *et al.* (1966), 68.7 to 94.5 per cent by Isshiki *et al.* (1967), and 68 to 114 per cent by Yoshioka *et al.* (1977). Therefore, PQ is usually larger than MFR during maximum sustained phonation (MFR = PV/MPT).

Hirano *et al.* (1968) demonstrated a highly positive relationship between MFR measured during maximum sustained phonation and PQ in normal subjects. They also reported that the PQ might prove a reasonable, clinical substitute for the MFR. The positive relationship between MFR measured during maximum sustained phonation and PQ was confirmed by Iwata and von Leden (1970) in pathological cases, and by Yoshioka *et al.* (1977) in normal and pathological subjects. The relationship between MFR measured during the phonation over a comfortable duration and PQ is not always significant (Shigemori, 1977; Yoshioka *et al.* 1977). One can measure PQ as a clinical substitute for MFR when no equipment for airflow measurement is available.

## 3. Normal Values of Phonation Quotient

Normal values of PQ in adults have been reported by several investigators (Table 3.8). The average PQ in the normal adult population seems to be between 120 and 190 ml/sec. The upper limit of the normal range varies between the different reports, ranging from 200 to 300 ml/sec.

Shigemori (1977) measured PQ of school children (Table 3.9). A large variation in PQ was observed among the children.

Table 3.8. *Normal values for phonation quotient (in ml/sec) in adults*

| Author(s) | N | | Average | Confidence limit | Critical region | Range |
|---|---|---|---|---|---|---|
| Sawashima (1966) | M | 50 | 139 | | 56—222 | |
| | F | 30 | 144 | | 66—222 | |
| Hirano *et al.* (1968) | M | 25 | 145 | 123—168 | 69—307 | |
| | F | 25 | 137 | 123—153 | 78—241 | |
| Shigemori (1977) | M | 25 | 145 | 125—169 | 67—314 | 72—328 |
| | F | 25 | 170 | 150—193 | 90—322 | 112—349 |
| Yoshioka *et al.* (1977) | M | 25 | 130 | | 56—205 | |
| | F | 25 | 126 | | 23—230 | |

Table 3.9. *Normal values for phonation quotient (in ml/sec) in school children (Shigemori, 1977)*

| Grade level | | Average | Confidence limit (95%) | Critical region (95%) | Range |
|---|---|---|---|---|---|
| 1st grade | male | 142 | 127—158 | 81—248 | 77—232 |
| | female | 143 | 126—162 | 75—272 | 63—226 |
| | total | 143 | 132—155 | 80—254 | 63—232 |
| 3rd grade | male | 165 | 149—182 | 98—276 | 107—235 |
| | female | 160 | 146—175 | 102—251 | 117—270 |
| | total | 162 | 152—173 | 102—259 | 107—270 |
| 5th grade | male | 177 | 164—192 | 119—264 | 114—244 |
| | female | 185 | 167—205 | 110—312 | 116—274 |
| | total | 182 | 170—194 | 115—286 | 114—274 |
| 7th grade | male | 209 | 177—246 | 91—482 | 103—463 |
| | female | 192 | 171—217 | 105—353 | 117—324 |
| | total | 201 | 182—221 | 99—406 | 103—463 |

## 4. Phonation Quotient in Pathological States

PQ in various laryngeal diseases was measured by Hirano *et al.* (1968), Iwata and von Leden (1972), Shigemori (1977) and Yoshioka *et al.* (1977). All the authors agree that PQ is markedly elevated in most cases of recurrent laryngeal nerve paralysis. Mass lesions of the vocal fold(s), including nodules, polyps, polypoid swelling and neoplasms, are often associated with an abnormally high PQ.

Shigemori (1977) reported that PQ is useful for monitoring the effect of surgical treatment in selected cases, especially in recurrent laryngeal nerve paralysis, and to some extent, in sulcus vocalis, and in cases with nodules, polyps or polypoid swelling.

# D. Subglottal Pressure

## 1. Technique of Measurement

### (1) Tracheal Puncture

A spinal needle or a modified version is inserted into the trachea through the cervical skin. It is connected to a pressure transducer or a manometer with a plastic tube. The frequency response of these systems is flat from 0 to 200 Hz at best. This technique has been adopted by many investigators (see Table 3.10) because of its validity. There are, however, two possible complications which can be serious: an injury to the esophagus and to the isthmus of the thyroid gland. They are usually avoided if the puncture is made at the cricothyroid space (cricothyroid space puncture).

### (2) Transglottal Catheter

A small catheter is inserted into the subglottal space through the mouth, the pharynx and the intercartilaginous portion of the glottis. It is connected to a pressure transducer or manometer. This technique is less invasive than the trachal puncture technique. However, it is occasionally difficult to keep the catheter from disturbing vocal fold vibration.

### (3) Measurement via a Tracheostoma

In those patients with tracheostomies, the subglottal pressure can be measured through the openings. However, such patients are few.

### (4) Esophageal Balloon

In contrast to the above methods, the esophageal balloon technique provides an indirect measurement. A balloon connected to a tube is inserted into the esophagus through the nose. The intratracheal pressure (approximately equal to subglottal pressure) is transmitted to the balloon via the posterior tracheal wall which is attached to the anterior esophageal wall. The intraesophageal pressure, measured in this way, does not represent the intratracheal pressure alone. The intratracheal pressure is a composite of the intraesophageal pressure and the pressure which is exerted by the elastic recoil of the lungs. The pressure produced by the elastic recoil of the lungs is positively related to the lung volume. Therefore, when the lung volume is high as after deep inspiration, the intraesophageal pressure is lower than the intratracheal pressure. On the contrary, when the lung volume is low as after forceful expiration, the intraesophageal pressure is higher than the intratracheal pressure. Thus, the estimation of the subglottal pressure from the intraesophageal pressure is valid only in some limited conditions.

### (5) Use of Transducer of Ultra-Miniature Type

An implantable ultra-miniature solid-state pressure transducer is directly placed in the subglottal space through the mouth, the pharynx and the intercartilaginous portion of the glottis. This technique was first reported by Koike and Perkins (1968). Because of its high frequency response (flat 0—20 KHz), the ultra-miniature pressure transducer allows us to register the pressure variations within one vibratory cycle. The greatest problem with this type of transducer lies in the fact that it is temperature-dependent.

## 2. Normal Values for Subglottal Pressure

Table 3.10 presents the normal values of subglottal pressure as reported by some investigators.

### (1) Habitual Phonation

In most cases, the subglottal pressure ($P_{SUB}$) during habitual phonation ranges from 5 to 10 cm $H_2O$, *i.e.* approximately 5.000 to 10.000 dyne/cm$^2$.

### (2) Variations in Vocal Intensity

It is generally agreed that $P_{SUB}$ is positively related to the vocal intensity. According to van den Berg (1956), the vocal intensity (I) is proportional to the fourth power of $P_{SUB}$ ($I \propto (P_{SUB})^4$). Isshiki (1964) reported that $I \propto (P_{SUB})^{3.3}$ in low pitch phonation, $I \propto (P_{SUB})^{3.3 \pm 0.7}$ in medium pitch phonation, and $I \propto (P_{SUB})^4$ or $I \propto (P_{SUB})^{3.3}$ in high pitch phonation.

### (3) Variations in Fundamental Frequency

Ohala (1970) measured rates of increase in fundamental frequency and $P_{SUB}$ when the muscular tension of the larynx is kept constant. His experiment involved having a subject maintain a steady pitch, and then pushing on the chest or abdomen at unexpected moments. $P_{SUB}$ was measured by the cricothyroid space puncture method. Activity of the laryngeal muscles was monitored electromyographically. The rate was 2—4 Hz/cm $H_2O$ for the modal voice and 7—10 Hz/cm $H_2O$ for falsetto.

Table 3.10. *Subglottal pressure (in cm H₂O) in normal subjects*

| Author(s) | Technique | Phonatory sample(s) | Subglottal pressure in cm $H_2O$ |
|---|---|---|---|
| Gutzmann and Loewy (1920) | Via tracheostoma | Vowel | Soft voice:        4.0— 5.0<br>Middle voice:  6.5—10.0<br>Loud voice:    14.0—23.0<br>Falsetto:          5.0—12.0 |
| van den Berg (1956) | Transglottal catheter<br>Esophageal balloon | Vowel | Chest (Soft-Loud):     5—11<br>Mid (Soft-Loud):       5—35<br>Falsetto (Soft-Loud): 6—50 |
| Isshiki (1959) | Tracheal puncture<br>Via tracheostoma | Vowel | 5—25 |
| Isshiki (1964) | Tracheal puncture | Vowel (with a cone in the mouth) | Low pitch:        4—10<br>Medium pitch: 4—25<br>High pitch:        7—22 |
| Kunze (1964) | Tracheal puncture | Vowel | 2.75—9.71 |
| Loebell (1969) | Tracheal puncture (cricothyroid space) | Vowel | Habitual phonation: 6—7<br>Loud phonation:      up to 26 |
| Ohala (1970) | Tracheal puncture (cricothyroid space) | Vowel | Low pitch (Soft-Loud):        5— 9<br>Medium pitch (Soft-Loud):  7—12<br>High pitch (Soft-Loud):        5—18<br>Falsetto (Soft-Loud):         10—16 |
| Yano (1963) | Tracheal puncture | Monosyllables | 3— 5 |
| Ladefoged and McKinny (1963) | Esophageal balloon | Monosyllable words<br>Vowel | 8—40 |
| Hiroto (1966) | Tracheal puncture<br>Via tracheotomy | Monosyllables | 2— 8 |
| Kuroki (1969) | Tracheal puncture<br>Via tracheotomy | Monosyllables | 8—20 |
| Draper *et al.* (1959) | Esophageal balloon | Series of syllables<br>Counting | Quiet talking:      2<br>Loud talking:      5<br>Shouting:           9<br>Loud shouting: 30 |
| Ladefoged (1960) | Tracheal puncture<br>Esophageal balloon | Sentences | 10 |
| Lieberman (1968) | Tracheal catheter<br>Esophageal balloon | Sentences | 5—10 |

In actual speech or singing, no consistent involvement of $P_{SUB}$ in regulating fundamental frequency has been reported.

*(4) Variation in Vocal Register*

No consistent differences in $P_{SUB}$ between different vocal registers have been demonstrated.

## 3. Subglottal Pressure in Pathological States

Table 3.11 shows $P_{SUB}$ in pathological cases. In carcinoma of the larynx, $P_{SUB}$ is always much higher than in normal subjects. Recurrent laryngeal nerve paralysis tends to be associated with high $P_{SUB}$. In laryngocele, $P_{SUB}$ is higher than in normal. Functional dysphonia can be accompanied by very high $P_{SUB}$.

Table 3.11. *Subglottal pressure (in cm $H_2O$) in pathological states*

| Author(s) | Technique | Phonatory sample(s) | Subglottal pressure in cm $H_2O$ | |
|---|---|---|---|---|
| Hiroto (1966) | Tracheal puncture Via tracheostoma | Monosyllables | Carcinoma (N = 4) | 45— 55 |
| | | | Recurrent nerve paralysis (N = 4) | 15— 17 |
| Kuroki (1969) | Tracheal puncture Via tracheostoma | Monosyllables | Recurrent nerve paralysis | |
| | | | unilateral (N = 4) | 4— 21 |
| | | | bilateral (N = 2) | 21— 47 |
| | | | Carcinoma (N = 5) | 31— 80 |
| | | | After partial laryngectomy (N = 4) | 31—101 |
| Loebell (1969) | Tracheal puncture (cricothyroid space) | Vowel Sentences | Functional dysphonia (N = 25) | up to 90 |
| | | | Carcinoma (N = 20) | 20— 80 |
| | | | Laryngocele (N = 2) | 20— 25 |

# E. Glottal Resistance

The glottal resistance (GR) cannot be measured directly. It is calculated by dividing $P_{SUB}$ by MFR. Isshiki (1964) reported that GR was 20—100 dyne sec/cm⁵ at low and medium pitches and 150 dyne sec/cm⁵ at high pitches. He also described that GR was positively related to vocal intensity at low and medium pitches, but did not vary significantly with the vocal intensity at high pitches.

The clinical application of GR awaits further investigation.

# References

Aron, E. (1892): Über einen Versuch, die Spannung der Luft in der Trachea des lebenden Menschen zu messen. Virchows Archiv für Path. Anat. und Physiol. und für Klin. Med. *129*, 426—435.

Bastian, H. J., Susam, R., Unger, E. (1978): Aerodynamic evaluation of the efficiency and functional diagnosis of the normal female voice. Folia Phoniat. *30*, 85—92.

Becher, R. (1973): Messungen von Atemgrößen als eine Methode zur Objektivierung der stimmlichen Leistungsfähigkeit. Dipl.-Arbeit, Berlin, Charité.

Beckett, R. L. (1971): The respirometer as a diagnostic and clinical tool in the speech clinic. J. Sp. Hear. Dis. *36*, 235—240.

Campbell, C. J., Murtagh, J., Raber, C. F. (1963): Laryngeal resistance to air flow. Ann. Otol. Rhinol. Laryngol. *72*, 5—30.

Draper, M. H., Ladefoged, P., Whitteridge, D. (1959): Respiratory muscles in speech. J. Sp. Hear. Res. *2*, 16—27.

Draper, M. H., Ladefoged, P., Whitteridge, D. (1960): Expiratory pressure and air flow during speech. Brit. Med. J. *1*, 1837–1843.

Edmons, T. D., Lilly, D. J., Hardy, J. C. (1971): Dynamic characteristics of air-pressure measuring systems used in speech research. J. Acoust. Soc. Amer. *50*, 1051–1057.

Faaborg-Andersen, K., Yanagihara, N., von Leden, H. (1967): Vocal pitch and intensity regulation. Arch. Otolaryngol. *85*, 447–454.

Ferris, B. G. jr., Mead, J., Opie, L. H. (1964): Partitioning respiratory flow resistance in man. J. Appl. Physiol. *19*, 653–658.

Fry, D. L., Stead, W. W., Ebert, R. V., Lubin, R. I., Wells, H. S. (1952): The measurement of intraesophageal pressure and its regulationship to intrathoracic pressure. J. Lab. Clin. Med. *40*, 664–673.

Gordon, M. T., Morton, F. M., Simpson, I. C. (1978): Air flow measurements in diagnosis assessment and treatment of mechanic dysphonia. Folia Phoniat. *30*, 161–174.

Gutzmann, H., Loewy, A. (1920): Über den intrapulmonalen Druck und den Luftverbrauch bei der normalen Atmung, bei phonetischen Vorgängen und bei der exspiratorischen Dyspnoe. Pflügers Arch. Ges. Physiol. *180*, 111–137.

Hast, M. H. (1961): Subglottic air pressure and neural stimulation in phonation. J. Appl. Physiol. *16*, 1142–1146.

Hardy, J. C., Edmonds, T. D. (1968): Electronic integrator for measurement of patients of the lung volume. J. Sp. Hear. Res. *11*, 777–786.

Hirano, M. (1970): Regulatory mechanism of voice in singing. (16-mm-Film.)

Hirano, M. (1975): Phonosurgery. Basic and clinical investigations. Otologia (Fukuoka) *21*, 239–440.

Hirano, M., Koike, Y., von Leden, H. (1968): Maximum phonation time and air usage during phonation. Folia Phoniat. *20*, 185–201.

Hirano, H., Miyahara, T., Hirose, H., Kiritani, S., Fujiyama, O. (1970): Airflow rate in singing. Annual Bulletin, Research Inst. Logoped. Phoniat. Univ. of Tokyo *4*, 55–66.

Hiroto, I. (1966): Mechanism of phonation. Pathophysiological aspects of the larynx. Pract. Otol. (Kyoto) *39*, 229–291.

Hyatt, R. E., Wilcox, R. E. (1961): Extrathoratic airway resistance in man. J. Appl. Physiol. *16*, 326–330.

Isshiki, N. (1959): Regulatory mechanism of the pitch and volume of voice. Pract. Otol. (Kyoto) *52*, 1065–1094.

Isshiki, N. (1964): Regulatory mechanism of vocal intensity variation. J. Sp. Hear. Res. *7*, 17–29.

Isshiki, N. (1965a): Phonation and airflow. Jpn. J. Logoped. Phoniat. *6*, 19–22.

Isshiki, N. (1965b): Vocal intensity and air flow rate. Folia Phoniat. *17*, 92–104.

Isshiki, N. (1969): Remarks on mechanism for vocal intensity variation. J. Sp. Hear. Res. *12*, 669 to 672.

Isshiki, N. (1977): Functional surgery of the larynx. (Official report at the 78th Annual Convention of the Oto-Rhino-Laryngological Society of Japan, Fukuoka.)

Isshiki, N., Okamura, H., Morimoto, M. (1967): Maximum phonation time and air flow rate during phonation: Simple clinical tests for vocal function. Ann. Otol. *76*, 998–1007.

Isshiki, N., von Leden, H. (1964): Hoarseness aerodynamic studies. Arch. Otolaryngol. *80*, 206–213.

Iwata, S., von Leden, H. (1970a): Clinical evaluation of vocal velocity index in laryngeal disease. Ann. Otol. Rhinol. Laryngol. *79*, 259–268.

Iwata, S., von Leden, H. (1970b): Phonation quotient in patients with laryngeal diseases. Folia Phoniat. *22*, 117–128.

Iwata, S., von Leden, H., Williams, D. (1972): Air flow measurement during phonation. J. Commun. Disord. *5*, 67–79.

Iwata, S., Esaki, T., Iwami, K., Mimura, Y. (1976): Air flow studies in the patients with laryngeal diseases during phonation. J. Nagoya Cy Univ. Med. Ass. *26*, 398–406.

Iwata, S., Esaki, T., Iwami, K., Takasu, T. (1976): Laryngeal function in patients with laryngeal polyps after laryngomicrosurgery. Pract. Otol. (Kyoto) *69*, 499–506.

Kitajima, K., Isshiki, N., Tanabe, M. (1978): Use of a hot-wire flow meter in study of laryngeal function. Studia Phonologica (Kyoto) *12*, 25–30.

Kolman, A. W., Gordon, M. T., Simpson, I. C., Morton, F. M. (1975): Assessment of vocal function by air-flow measurements. Folia Phoniat. *27*, 250–262.

Klingholz, F., Siegert, C. (1972): Beziehungen zwischen Stimm-Schalldruck und intrathorakalem Druck beim Stimmeinsatz. Folia Phoniat. *24*, 381–386.

Knowles, J. H., Hong, S. K., Raph, H. (1959): Possible errors using esophageal balloon in determination of pressure-volume characteristics of the lung and thoracic cage. J. Appl. Physiol. *14*, 525—530.

Koike, Y. (1969): A method for direct determination of subglottal pressure. J. Acoust. Soc. Amer. *46*, 96—107.

Koike, Y., Hirano, M. (1968): Significance of vocal velocity index. Folia Phoniat. *20*, 285—296.

Koike, Y., Hirano, M., von Leden, H. (1967): Vocal initation; Acoustic and aerodynamic investigation on normal subjects. Folia Phoniat. *19*, 173—182.

Koike, Y., Perkins, W. H. (1968): Application of a miniaturized pressure transducer for experimental speech research. Folia Phoniat. *20*, 360—368.

Koike, Y., von Leden, H. (1969): Pathologic vocal initiation. Ann. Otol. Rhinol. Laryngol. *78*, 138—148.

Kunze, L. E. (1964): Evaluation of methods of estimating subglottal air pressure. J. Sp. Hear. Res. *7*, 151—164.

Kuroki, K. (1969): Subglottic pressure of normal and pathological larynges. Otologia (Fukuoka) *15*, 54—74.

Ladefoged, P. (1960): The regulation of subglottal pressure. Folia Phoniat. *12*, 169—175.

Ladefoged, P. (1962): Sub-glottal activity during speech in Sovijarvi and Aalto. Proc. 4th Int. Congr. of Phonetic Science, 73.

Ladefoged, P. (1964): Comment on evaluation of methodes of estimating subglottal air pressure. J. Sp. Hear. Res. *7*, 291—292.

Ladefoged, P., McKinney, N. P. (1963): Loudness, sound pressure, and subglottal pressure in speech. J. Acoust. Soc. Amer. *35*, 454—460.

Large, J., Iwata, S. (1971): Aerodynamic study of vibrato and voluntary "Straight tone" pairs in singing. Folia Phoniat. *23*, 50—65.

Large, J., Iwata, S., von Leden, H. (1970): The primary female register transition in singing. Folia Phoniat. *22*, 385—396.

Large, J., Iwata, S., von Leden, H. (1972): The male operatic head register versus falsetto. Folia Phoniat. *24*, 19—29.

Lieberman, P. (1968): Direct comparison of subglottal and esophageal pressure during speech. J. Acous. Soc. Amer. *43*, 1157—1164.

Löebell, E. (1969): Über die direkte Messung des subglottischen Luftdrucks. Arch. Ohr-Nas.-Kehlkheilkd. *194*, 316—320.

Maekawa, H., Kitabatake, S., Itoh, M., Watanabe, T., Simizu, T. (1975): The phonation quotient and the expiratory expenditure index in normal children. Jpn. J. Logop. Phoniat. *16*, 63—75.

McGlone, R. E. (1966): An investigation of air flow and subglottal air pressure related to fundamental frequency of phonation. Folia Phoniat. *18*, 312—322.

McGlone, R. E. (1967): Air flow during vocal fry phonation. J. Sp. Hear. Res. *10*, 299—304.

McGlone, R. E. (1967): Intraesophageal air pressure during syllable repetition. J. Acoust. Soc. Amer. *42*, 1280 A.

Milic-Emili, J., Mead, J., Turner, J. M., Glauser, E. M. (1964): Improved technique for estimating pleural pressure from esophageal balloons. J. Appl. Physiol. *19*, 207—216.

Murry, T. (1971): Subglottal pressure and airflow measures during vocal fry phonation. J. Sp. Hear. Res. *14*, 544—551.

Murry, T., Brown, W. S., jr. (1971): Subglottal air pressure during two types of vocal activity; Vocal fry and modal phonation. Folia Phoniat. *23*, 440—449.

Murry, T., Schmitke, L. K. (1975): Air flow onset and variability. Folia Phoniat. *27*, 401—409.

Nishida, Y., Suwowa, H. (1964): Indirect measuring method of subglottic pressure in the voice production, intraoesophageal method and interruption method. Otologia (Fukuoka) *10*, 264—270.

Perkins, W. H., Koike, Y. (1969): Patterns of subglottal pressure variations during phonation. A preliminary report. Folia Phoniat. *21*, 1—8.

Rothenberg, M. (1973): A new inverse-filtering technique for deriving the glottal air flow waveform during voicing. J. Acoust. Soc. Amer. *53*, 1632—1645.

Rubin, H. J. (1963): Experimental studies on vocal pitch and intensity in phonation. Laryngoscope *73*, 973—1015.

Rubin, H. J., Hills, B., Lecover, M., Vennard, W. (1967): Vocal intensity, subglottic pressure and air flow relationship in singers. Folia Phoniat. *19*, 393—413.

Saito, S. (1977): Phonosurgery. Basic study on the mechanism of phonation and endolaryngeal microsurgery. Otologia (Fukuoka) *23*, 171—384.

Sawashima, M. (1966): Measurement of maximum phonation time. Jpn. J. Logoped. Phoniat. *7*, 23—28.

Schilder, D. P., Hyatt, R. E., Fry, D. L. (1959): An improved balloon system for measuring intraesophageal pressure. J. Appl. Physiol. *14*, 1057—1058.

Schwabe, F., Siegert, C. (1973): Bemerkungen zum Beitrag "Vocal intensity, subglottic pressure and air
flow relationships in singers". Folia Phoniat. *25*, 150—154.

Sehilling, R. (1925): Untersuchungen über die Atembewegungen beim Sprechen und Singen. Mschr.
Ohrenheilk. Laryngo-Rhinol. *59*, 643—668.

Shigemori, Y. (1977): Some tests related to the air usage during phonation. Clinical investigations.
Otologia (Fukuoka) *23*, 138—166.

Smith, S. (1959): Le jet d'air relatif aux mouvements des corders vocalis des deux modèles. J. F. O. R. *8*,
113—118.

Smith, S. (1960): The electro-areometer. Speech Path. Ther. 28—29.

Strenger, F. (1960): Methods for direct and indirect measurement of the subglottic air pressure in phonation. Studia Linguistica *14*, 98—112.

Suzuki, T. (1944): Investigations of expiratory air volume during phonation. Tohoku Med. J. *34*,
93—104.

Unger, E., Bastian, H.-J., Sasama, R. (1975): Aerodynamische Leistungsprüfung und Funktionsdiagno-
stik der normalen Frauenstimme. (Vortr. 5, Phoniatriesymposion, Leipzig.)

Utenick, M. R. (1971): Design of a hot anemometer. ISA Transact. *10*, 21—28.

van den Berg, Jw. (1956): Direct and Indirect determination of the mean subglottic pressure. Folia
Phoniat. *8*, 1—24.

van den Berg, Jw. (1957): Subglottic pressures and vibrations of the vocal folds. Folia Phoniat. *9*, 65—71.

Watanabe, Y., Hirano, M., Matsushita, H., Kawasaki, H., Shigemori, Y. (1975): Air usage during phonation in normal school children. Jpn. J. Logoped. Phoniat. *16*, 1—5.

Worth, J. H., Runyon, J. C., Subtelny, J. D. (1968): Integrating flowmeter for measuring unimpaired oral
and nasal airflow. IEEE Transact. on Bio-Med. Eng. *15*, 196—200.

Yanagihara, N., Koike, Y. (1967): The regulation of sustained phonation. Folia Phoniat. *19*, 1—18.

Yanagihara, N., Koike, Y., von Leden, H. (1967): Respiration and phonation—The functional examination of laryngeal disease. Folia Phoniat. *19*, 153—166.

Yanagihara, N., von Leden, H. (1966): Phonation and Respiration. Function study in normal subjects.
Folia Phoniat. *18*, 323—340.

Yano, T. (1963): Studies on the air pressure in the vocal tract during phonation. Pract. Otol. (Kyoto) *56*,
531—561.

Yoshioka, H., Sawashima, M., Hirose, H., Ushijima, T., Honda, K. (1977): Clinical evaluation of air
usage during phonation. Jpn. J. Logoped. Phoniat. *18*, 87—93.

Yoshiya, I., Nakajima, T., Nagai, I., Jitsukawa, S. (1975): A bidirectional respiratory flowmeter using the
hot-wire principle. J. Appl. Physiol. *38*, 360—365.

# Examination of Vocal Fold Vibration  4

## A. General Description

### 1. Methods of Examination of Vocal Fold Vibration

The vocal folds usually vibrate at 100–300 Hz during normal conversation, and even at 1000 Hz or more during singing. Observation of such vibrations requires special methods. The following methods are available at present.

(1) Stroboscopy
(2) Ultra high speed photography
(3) Photo-electric glottography
(4) Electroglottography
(5) Ultrasound glottography

Stroboscopy is the most useful for clinical purpose. Ultra high speed photography has been employed chiefly for research and educational purposes. The apparatus is too expensive and the data processing is too time-consuming for most clinicians. Vibration of the vocal fold itself is not directly viewed with the glottographies, although they provide some information about vocal fold vibration. A great advantage of glottography is that immediate graphic displays of the results can be obtained. Details of each technique will be described later in this chapter.

### 2. Parameters to Be Assessed in Vocal Fold Vibration

*(1) Horizontal Excursion of the Edge of the Vocal Fold(s) (Fig. 4.2A)*

The term "edge" means the part of the vocal fold which is located most medially. The edge is not a fixed part of the vocal fold. The innermost part of the vocal fold varies within each vibratory cycle (see Fig. 4.1). The edge of the vocal fold also moves in vertical and longitudinal directions, but it is difficult to quantify the movements in these directions.

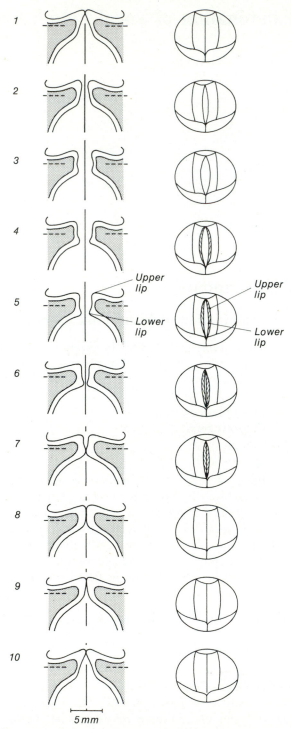

Fig. 4.1. Schematic presentation of vocal fold vibration. Left column: frontal section, right column: view from above

## (2) Glottal Width (Fig. 4.2B)

The term glottal width means the distance between the edges of the vocal folds in a given frontal plane.

## (3) Glottal Area (Fig. 4.2C)

The area surrounded by the edges of the vocal folds is called the glottal area. In the normal vibration, the glottal area waveform resembles the glottal width waveform determined at the middle of the membraneous part. The glottal area waveform is similar to the volume velocity waveform, but there is some difference between these two waveforms.

## (4) Fundamental Frequency or Fundamental Period of Vibration

The time span required for one vibratory cycle is called the fundamental period. The fundamental frequency ($F_0$) and the fundamental period (P) are related as:

$$F_0 \times P = 1$$

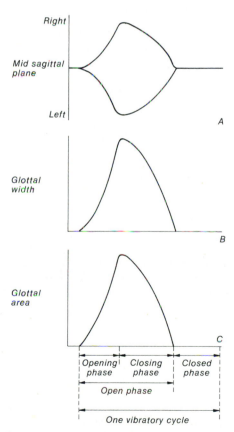

Fig. 4.2. Phases in one vibratory cycle. *A* Horizontal excursion, *B* Glottal width, *C* Glottal area

*(5) Opening Phase, Closing Phase, Open Phase and Closed Phase*

One vibratory cycle is divided into two major phases: the open phase and the closed phase. The open phase is further divided into the opening and closing phases (Fig. 4.2).

*(6) Open Quotient (OQ), Speed Quotient (SQ) and Speed Index (SI)*

The open quotient (OQ) is defined as:

$$OQ = \frac{\tau \text{ (open phase)}}{\tau \text{ (entire cycle)}}$$

where

$\tau$ (open phase) = duration of the open phase,
$\tau$ (entire cycle) = duration of the entire cycle
or fundamental period.

The larger the open phase, the larger the OQ. The value of OQ is one when there is no complete glottal closure.

The speed quotient (SQ) is defined as:

$$SQ = \frac{\tau \text{ (opening phase)}}{\tau \text{ (closing phase)}} = \frac{\text{average speed of closing}}{\text{average speed of opening}}$$

where

$\tau$ (opening phase) = duration of the opening phase,
$\tau$ (closing phase) = duration of the closing phase.

The speed index (SI) is defined as:

$$SI = \frac{\tau \text{(opening phase)} - \tau \text{ (closing phase)}}{\tau \text{(opening phase)} + \tau \text{ (closing phase)}}$$

$$= \frac{SQ - 1}{SQ + 1}$$

Table 4.1 represents the relationship between SQ and SI. SI seems to be advantageous over SQ for the following reasons: (1) SI ranges from $-1$ to 1 whereas SQ ranges over large values. (2) When two waveforms have the same triangular shape and one is the reverse of the other (with respect to time), the SI takes equal absolute values with reverse signs. On the other hand, the SQ takes two different values whose product is 1. (3) One can visualize the waveform from SI values more easily than from SQ values. (4) SI has a simpler relationship with the spectral characteristics of the waveform than SQ.

*(7) Amplitude*

The size of the greatest displacement is called the maximum amplitude or simply the amplitude.

Table 4.1. *Comparison of SQ and SI. The triangles present the waveforms when SI is −1.00, 0.00 and 1.00, respectively*

| Opening | : | Closing | SQ | SI |
|---|---|---|---|---|
| 0 | : | 10 | 0.00 | −1.00 |
| 1 | : | 9 | 0.11 | −0.80 |
| 2 | : | 8 | 0.25 | −0.60 |
| 3 | : | 7 | 0.43 | −0.40 |
| 4 | : | 6 | 0.67 | −0.20 |
| 5 | : | 5 | 1.00 | 0.00 |
| 6 | : | 4 | 1.50 | 0.20 |
| 7 | : | 3 | 2.33 | 0.40 |
| 8 | : | 2 | 4.00 | 0.60 |
| 9 | : | 1 | 9.00 | 0.80 |
| 10 | : | 0 | ∞ | 1.00 |

## (8) Regularity or Periodicity of Successive Vibrations

Cycle-to-cycle variations of the fundamental period, the amplitude and/or the waveform are to be examined.

## (9) Symmetry of the Bilateral Vocal Folds

Symmetrical movements of the vocal folds indicate that their mechanical properties are the same. Differences in mechanical properties of the two vocal folds result in asymmetrical vibrations.

## (10) Homogeneity

The structure of the normal vocal fold is roughly homogenous along its longitudinal axis. Therefore, different points along the longitudinal axis, do not usually present substantial phase differences. The amplitude is usually largest at the middle of the membraneous portion.

## (11) Mucosal Wave

In the normal vocal fold, waves travelling on the mucosa from the inferior to its superior surface are observed during vibrations, except for falsetto. This wave is called mucosal wave or travelling wave on the mucosa. The speed of the wave is normally 0.5 to 1 m/sec. Existence of a soft and pliant superficial layer of the lamina propria is supposed to be essential for the occurrence of the mucosal wave.

## (12) Upper Lip and Lower Lip

At certain phases during each vibratory cycle, two lip-like eminences are observed near the edge of the vocal fold. They are called upper and lower lips. They are usually best observed immediately after maximum opening of the vocal folds (Fig. 4.1). During the opening phase, the lower lip is covered by the upper lip and, therefore, is not viewed from above. The edge of the vocal fold represents mainly the upper lip. During the closing phase, the two lips are usually observable from above. The closed phase typically begins with an approximation of the lower lips. The edge of the vocal fold, therefore, represents mainly the lower lip during the closing phase. In the closed phase, the upper and lower lips become indistinguishable.

The upper and lower lips are not definite portions of a vocal fold. The locations where these eminences occur vary within each vibratory cycle.

### (13) Contact Area of the Vocal Folds

During the closed phase, the contact area of the bilateral vocal folds changes with time. This cannot be observed from above. In electroglottography and ultrasound glottography, information about the contact area is reflected in the output signals.

## 3. Three Typical Vibratory Patterns of Normal Vocal Folds

Normal vocal folds present three typical vibratory patterns: that for falsetto, that for modal voice and that for vocal fry (Fig. 4.3). In the falsetto, no complete glottic closure takes place ($OQ = 1$). The modal voice is associated with a complete glottic closure ($OQ < 1$). In the vocal fry, the closed phase is very long relative to the entire period and there are occasionally two open phases during one vibratory cycle (Moore and von Leden, 1958).

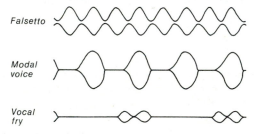

Fig. 4.3. Typical vibratory patterns of normal vocal folds

## B. Stroboscopy

Stroboscopic examination, as a routine clinical test, is the most practical technique for examination of the vibratory pattern of the vocal folds. It was as early as 1895 that a laryngo-stroboscope first came into use as a means of observing the normal vibration of the vocal folds (Oertel, 1895; Musehold, 1898). In the early stages, mechanical devices were adopted to obtain an intermittent source of light. It was, therefore, very difficult to examine pathological vibrations which were associated with irregular cycle-to-cycle variations. Application of a strobo-light bulb with an electronic device to the laryngo-stroboscope in the 1950's made it feasible to utilize the stroboscope for clinical purposes (Beck and Schönhärl, 1954; Timcke, 1956). Schönhärl (1960) first made pioneering and extensive investigations on modern laryngo-stroboscopy. Since then, stroboscopic examinations have become popular in many voice clinics.

## 1. Principle

The light source of the stroboscope emits intermittent flashes of light which are synchronous with the vibratory cycles. The source of the trigger signal for the light flashes is the waveform of the subject's voice. When the flashes are emitted at the same frequency as that of the vocal fold vibration, that is, at an identical phase point in successive vibratory cycles, a sharp and a clear image of the vocal folds is observed (Fig. 4.4A), assuming that the reappearance of the waveform is maintained constant. When the flashes are emitted at frequencies slightly less than the frequency of vocal fold vibration, giving rise to a systematic phase delay of the consecutive light flashes, a slow motion effect is produced (Fig. 4.4B).

Stroboscopy does not show fine details of each vibratory cycle, but it demonstrates a vibratory pattern averaged over many successive cycles. This is the essential difference between stroboscopy and ultra high speed photography.

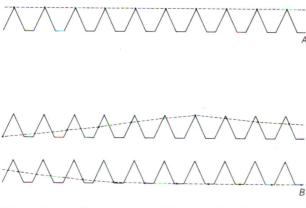

Fig. 4.4. Schematic presentation of the principle of stroboscopy

## 2. Apparatus

Several kinds of apparatus are available (Fig. 4.5). Basically, the apparatus consists of a microphone, a light source, an electronic control unit and a pedal. It has at least the following three functions: (1) To extract the fundamental period of the voice signal and to emit light flashes synchronous with the voice signal, (2) To vary the phase point when the light flashes, and (3) To indicate the fundamental frequency of phonation.

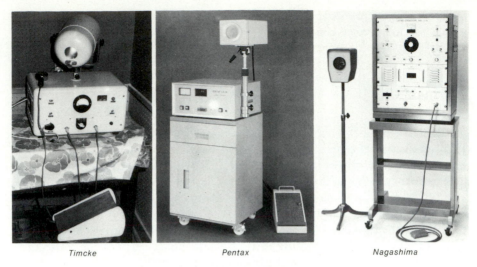

Timcke                    Pentax                    Nagashima

Fig. 4.5. Laryngo-stroboscopes


## 3. Items to Be Observed

It is recommended to observe and describe, at least, the following items:

*(1) Fundamental Frequency*

The fundamental frequency is read on the pitch indicator of the stroboscope. When it varies during the examination, the range of the variation should be described.

*(2) Symmetry of the Bilateral Movements*

One should first check to see if the movements of the vocal folds are symmetrical or not. If they are asymmetrical, it is advisable to describe how asymmetrical they are, for example, "The amplitude is greater on the right side than on the left", or "The excursion of the right vocal fold significantly lags behind that of the left vocal fold".

*(3) Regularity (Periodicity)*

The regularity of successive vibrations should be examined. The results are described with the term "regular (periodic)" or "irregular (aperiodic)".

*(4) Glottal Closure*

One should find out if complete glottal closure takes place during the vibratory cycles. When the glottis is completely closed, it is advisable to describe qualitatively the length of the closed phase as: "very long", "long", "fairly long", "short" or "very short". When the glottal closure is incomplete, it is advisable to draw the shape of the glottis at the maximum closing.

## (5) Amplitude

The maximum amplitude of the horizontal excursion of the vocal folds is determined subjectively and qualitatively. It is described as: "greater than normal", "normal", "smaller than normal", or "zero". Differences in the amplitude of the two vocal folds, if there are any, are also described.

## (6) Mucosal Wave

The size of the mucosal wave on the vocal folds is determined subjectively and qualitatively. It is described as: "greater than normal", "normal", "smaller than normal", or "none". Differences, if any, in the mucosal wave between the vocal folds are also described.

## (7) Non-Vibrating Portion

If there is any portion of the vocal fold which does not vibrate, in other words, which remains immobile during phonation, this should be specified. The absence of vibratory movement can occur either occasionally or always.

## (8) Others

If any other findings are made, it is advisable to describe them. For example: "The polyp moves with a delay from the vocal fold proper." "The edge of the right vocal fold crosses the midline toward the end of the medial excursion."

Table 4.2 present an example of a form of stroboscopic record.

Table 4.2. *A form for the record of stroboscopic findings (Hirano, 1975)*

Stroboscopic findings:

1. Fundamental frequency _____ Hz.
2. Symmetry
   (1) symmetrical
   (2) asymmetrical     i · in amplitude (+, −) (R ≷ L)
                          ii · in phase      (+, −)
3. Regularity (periodicity)
   (1) regular
   (2) irregular
   (3) inconsistent (sometimes regular, sometimes irregular)
4. Glottic closure
   (1) complete
   (2) incomplete
   (3) inconsistent (sometimes complete, sometimes incomplete)
5. Amplitude
   Right (1) great (2) normal (3) small (4) zero
   Left   (1) great (2) normal (3) small (4) zero
6. Wave
   Right (1) great (2) normal (3) small (4) absent
   Left   (1) great (2) normal (3) small (4) absent
7. Non-vibrating portion
   Right (1) none (2) occasionally, partially (3) always, partially (4) occasionally, entirely
           (5) always, entirely
   Left   (1) none (2) occasionally, partially (3) always, partially (4) occasionally, entirely
           (5) always, entirely
8. Other findings
   (1) none (2) noted

4 *

# 4. Instruction Notes

*(1) Practice*

Since the stroboscopic observations depend on subjective evaluations of the examiner, one has to practice so as to be capable of making accurate observations. Repeated observations of normal subjects phonating at different fundamental frequencies and at different intensities provide the examiner with a rough guide about normal variations. The viewing of ultra high speed films of normal and pathological conditions is also very helpful.

*(2) Variations of the Vibratory Pattern Depending on the Manner of Phonation*

There are the following general tendencies:

(i) As the fundamental frequency increases, the amplitude of vibration and the mucosal wave decrease and the closed phase becomes relatively shorter, assuming that the vocal effort is roughly constant.

(ii) As the vocal intensity increases, the amplitude and the mucosal wave increase and the closed phase becomes relatively longer.

(iii) In falsetto, the amplitude is small, the mucosal wave is hardly found, and the glottis is not completely closed.

*(3)* Some patients tend not to phonate normally when they are examined by indirect laryngoscopy. The examiner should therefore carefully note the manner in which the patient phonates during the examination. He should instruct the patient to try to phonate under relaxed conditions. If there is any difference in phonation during stroboscopy from that under relaxed conditions, describe the manner of phonation during the examination, for example, "The voice was strained during stroboscopy", or "The pitch was higher during stroboscopy than in normal conversation".

# 5. Some Notes Relevant to Interpretation of Findings

In interpreting stroboscopic findings, it is helpful to understand the effects of various factors on the observations made.

*(1) Fundamental Frequency*

(a) As the vibrating portion of the vocal fold becomes shorter, the fundamental frequency increases.

(b) The stiffer the vocal fold, the greater the fundamental frequency.

(c) As the mass of the vocal fold increases, the fundamental frequency decreases.

(d) The greater the subglottal pressure, the greater the fundamental frequency.

*(2) Symmetry*

If there are any differences in the mechanical properties, for example the position, shape, mass, elasticity and viscosity, of the vocal folds, their vibratory movements become asymmetrical.

*(3) Periodicity*

Maintenance of periodical vibrations of a vibrator calls for a steady balance between the mechanical properties of the vibrator and the force applied to the vibrator. The following conditions can impair this balance, and result in aperiodical vibrations:

(a) Marked asymmetry in the mechanical properties of the vocal folds.
(b) Marked interference with the homogeneity of the vocal fold(s).
(c) Incapability of maintaining a steady tonus of the laryngeal muscles.
(d) Incapability of blowing out the air from the lungs with a consistent force.

*(4) Glottal Closure*

An incomplete glottal closure during vocal fold vibration can result from the following:

(a) An impaired adduction of the vocal fold(s).
(b) A non-linear edge of the vocal fold(s).
(c) Any obstacle intervening between the two vocal folds.
(d) A stiff edge of the vocal fold(s).

*(5) Amplitude*

(a) The shorter the vibrating portion of the vocal folds, the smaller the amplitude.
(b) The stiffer the vocal fold, the smaller the amplitude.
(c) As the mass of the vocal fold increases, the amplitude decreases.
(d) The existence of an obstacle results in a decrease of amplitude.
(e) As the subglottal pressure increases, the amplitude becomes greater.

*(6) Mucosal Wave*

(a) The stiffer the mucosa, the less marked the mucosal wave.
(b) When the mucosa is only partially stiff, the wave stops travelling at the stiff portion.
(c) The greater the subglottal pressure, the more marked the mucosal wave.

## 6. Optional Devices

*(1) Stroboscopic Examination Under Microscopy*

With the use of stroboscopic light for illumination during endolaryngeal microscopy, vibration of the vocal folds can be observed at a magnification. Vibratory behavior of different portions of the vocal folds are examined in detail. Neuroleptanalgesia without intratracheal intubation is required so that the subject can phonate with a laryngoscope in his throat. Saito (1977) used this technique to monitor the immediate results of surgery.

Pascher *et al.* (1971), Seidner *et al.* (1972) and Padovan *et al.* (1973) used an operation microscope and a laryngeal mirror for stroboscopic observation in the consulting room.

*(2) Use of Fiberscope*

For those subjects whose vocal folds are not visualized under a laryngeal mirror, a fiberscope connected to a stroboscopic light is useful. Apparatuses for the fiberoptic stroboscopy have been developed by Saito (1977) and Yoshida *et al.* (1977).

*(3) Cinematography and Video-Tape Recording of Stroboscopic Images*

One of the shortcomings of stroboscopy was the difficulty in keeping a record of the images observed. Saito (1977) and Yoshida *et al.* (1979) developed systems for cinematography and/or video-tape recording which are easily utilized in office clinics. Such devices are valuable, especially, for the following reasons:

(1) The physician can use not only verbal but also visual means to explain the laryngeal condition to the patients.

(2) Teaching the various aspects of vocal fold vibration can be enhanced with the use of this dynamic method.

(3) More accurate information can be gleaned by allowing more than one specialist to view the vocal fold in motion at the same time. In addition, this system permits repeated viewings at convenient times.

(4) One can compare vibratory patterns at different times including pre- and post-therapeutic examinations.

# C. Ultra High Speed Photography

In 1937, scientists at the Bell Telephone Laboratories succeeded in photographing the vibrating human vocal folds at ultra high speeds. Since then, several investigators have reported their own techniques (Dunker and Schlosshauer, 1958; Tsuiki *et al.*, 1958; Luchsinger and Pfister, 1959; Sonesson, 1960; Le Cover and Rubin, 1960; Moore and von Leden, 1962; Moore *et al.*, 1962; von Leden *et al.*, 1966; Hiroto *et al.*, 1966; Dubovik, 1968; Hirano, Yoshida *et al.*, 1974). Frame-by-frame analysis investigations of ultra high speed films have produced an incredible amount of information about the behavior of the vocal folds in normal and pathological conditions (Timcke *et al.*, 1958; Moore and von Leden, 1958; Timcke *et al.*, 1959; von Leden *et al.*, 1960; Rubin and Hirt, 1960; von Leden and Moore, 1961; Isshiki and von Leden, 1963/1964; von Leden and Isshiki, 1965; Hiroto, 1966; Yoshida, 1969; Hirano, 1970; Hirano *et al.*, 1971; Hirano *et al.*, 1973; Koike and Hirano, 1973; Hirano, Matsushita *et al.*, 1974; Hirano, 1975; Kawasaki, 1976; Kakita *et al.*, 1976a, 1976b; Hirano *et al.*, 1978; Kobayashi, 1978).

## 1. Principle

The vibrating vocal folds are photographed with a number of frames at a rate which is about 20 to 30 times the fundamental frequency of the phonation. For example, if the vocal folds, vibrating at 120 Hz, are photographed at a film speed of 3.000 frames per second, images of 25 phase points are photographed within one vibratory cycle (Fig. 4.6). When one views this film running at a normal speed (24

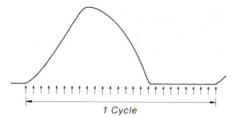

*1 Cycle*

Fig. 4.6. Schematical presentation of the principle of ultra high speed photography

frames per second), the events are observed in an ultra slow motion. The time dimension is expanded by 125 times. Frame-by-frame analysis of various parameters demonstrates the vibratory behavior in detail.

## 2. Apparatus

The apparatus for ultra high speed photography basically consists of an extremely bright light source; an optical system to reflect light from the subject's larynx to a camera unit; an ultra high speed camera; an electric or electronic system to operate the light source and the camera; and a pulse generator which provides time marks. Fig. 4.7 schematically shows the system devised by Hirano, Yoshida *et al.* (1974).

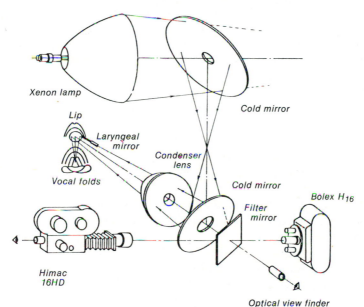

Fig. 4.7. Schematical presentation of a system for ultra high speed photography of the vocal folds
(Hirano *et al.*, 1974)

## 3. Application

Ultra high speed photography requires an expensive apparatus. Furthermore, the data processing is very time-consuming. For these reasons, it has not been applied clinically. It is, however, extremely useful for research and teaching purposes.

# D. Photo-Electric Glottography

Glottal area variation can be recorded with the use of a photo-electric device which converts light intensity into electrical voltage. The glottis is illuminated from above or below and the intensity of the light passing through the glottis is measured with a light sensor placed on the opposite side (relative to the position of the light source).

Sonneson (1959, 1960) first used this device on the human larynx. In his technique, a bright DC light source is placed against the neck just below the larynx. The light suffuses through the subglottic space and transilluminates the glottis. A curved light-conducting rod is passed through the mouth and terminates at the level of the epiglottis. A photo-multiplier tube is connected to the oral end of the rod. Ohala (1966) incased a small light sensor in a transparent flexible plastic catheter. The light sensor is located 25 cm from the tip of the catheter. The catheter is inserted into the pharynx and the esophagus through the nose, so that the sensor faces the laryngeal aperture. A similar technique was also used by Frøkjaer-Jensen (1967). Sawashima (1968) and Lisker *et al.* (1969) reversed the positions of light source and photo-sensor relative to the glottis.

Sawashima (1968) inserted a flexible fiber-optic through the nose to obtain the transillumination record simultaneously with a motion picture of the larynx during speech. The light source for the laryngeal photography also served for the transillumination. A photo-multiplier tube was placed against the trachea just below the larynx. He noted that a shift of the level of output signal could be caused by moving the optical cable relative to the larynx and, hence, concluded that visual or photographic monitoring of the glottis was indispensable for the correct interpretation of the photo-electric glottogram.

Coleman and Wendal (1968) recorded photo-electric glottograms simultaneously with ultra high speed motion photography during sustained phonation. They found a significant difference between the glottal waveforms obtained by the two methods. They pointed out the following factors as possible sources of error in photo-electric glottography:

(1) The light-density distribution within the vocal folds may not be constant.

(2) The changing cross-sectional area of the vocal folds in an anterior-posterior plane may result in an uneven illumination of the folds.

(3) Light reflections from the mucosal surfaces may be variable.

(4) Vertical movements of the vocal folds towards and from the light source are not taken into account.

(5) The location of the monitoring device causes different waveforms.

For these reasons, Colman and Wendal concluded that, without acceptable validation of the procedures, the interpretation of photo-electric glottographic data ought to be regarded with scepticism, particularly when the spectral properties of the glottal wave are concerned.

# E. Electroglottography (Electrolaryngography)

Electroglottography makes use of motion-induced variations in the electrical impedance between two electrodes placed on the skin of the neck. The electrodes are placed above the thyroid laminae. A weak, high-frequency voltage of 0.5—10 MHz is applied to one electrode, and the other electrode picks up the electrical current passing through the larynx. The transverse electrical impedance varies with the opening and closing of the glottis, and results in a variation of the electrical current in phase with the vibratory phases of the vocal folds.

This technique was first reported by Fabre (1957). Improvements in the apparatus and application of the technique to basic and clinical investigations have been extensively performed mostly in Europe. (Chevrie-Muller, 1962, 1964, 1967; Fabre, 1958, 1961; Fant *et al.*, 1966; Fischer-Jørgensen *et al.*, 1966; Frøkjaer-Jensen, 1968; Frøkjaer-Jensen and Thorvaldsen, 1968; Fourcin and Norgate, 1965; Fourcin and West, 1968; Fourcin and Abberton, 1971; Fourcin, 1979; Gougerot *et al.*, 1960; Grémy, 1963; Holm, 1969, 1970, 1971; Köster and Smith, 1970; Lebrun, 1971; Lecluse *et al.*, 1975; Lecluse, 1976, 1977 a, 1977 b; Loebell, 1968, 1970; Neil *et al.*, 1977; Striglioni, 1963; Vallancien and Faulhaber, 1967; Vallancien *et al.*, 1971; van Michel, 1964, 1966, 1967; van Michel and Raskin, 1969; van Michel *et al.*, 1970).

Lecluse and his co-workers (1975, 1977) recorded electroglottograms simultaneously with stroboscopic images, and related the electroglottographic recordings to the glottal images viewed from above (Fig. 4.8).

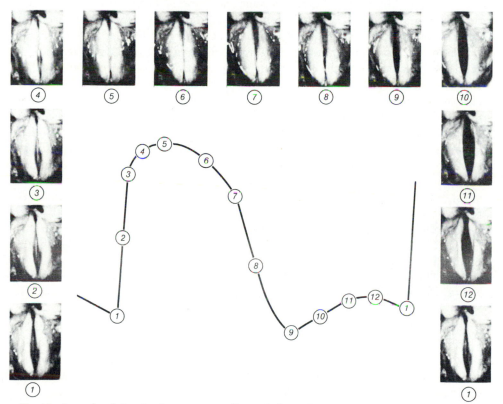

Fig. 4.8. A result of the simultaneous recordings of electroglottograms and stroboscopic images (Lecluse, 1977)

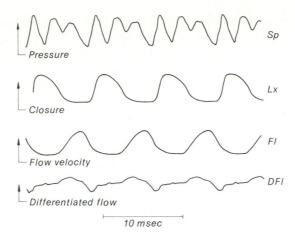

Fig. 4.9. Simultaneous recording of sound pressure *(Sp)*, electroglottogram *(Lx)*, airflow velocity *(Fl)* and time differential *(DFl)* of the airflow velocity (Fourcin, 1979)

Fourcin (1979) made simultaneous recordings of electroglottograms and airflow velocity curves for different modes of phonation, and described how to interprete the electrograms (Fig. 4.9). He also emphasized that the fundamental period of vocal fold vibration could be determined quite accurately on the electroglottogram.

In contrast to photo-electric glottography whose output signal reflects the size of the glottal area during the open phase, the output signal of electroglottography conveys information about the contact area of the vocal folds (for example, Köster and Smith, 1970). Therefore, electroglottography might be useful for investigating the glottal condition during the closed phase. The electroglottogram, however, appears to be considerably affected by artefacts, including variations in the impedance between the electrodes and the skin, vertical displacements of the larynx relative to the electrodes, condition of cervical structures other than the glottis, and so on. It is difficult to determine the extent to which the contact area of the vocal folds contributes to the output signal of electroglottography. At present, the following observations may be made on electroglottography:

(1) The procedure is associated with minimum discomfort to the subject.

(2) The electroglottogram reflects the glottal condition better during the closed phase than during the open phase.

(3) The presence or absence of glottal vibrations can be readily determined.

(4) The fundamental period of vibration is easily determined as the beginning of each closed phase is marked by a sharp rise in the graphic display.

(5) Quantitative interpretation of the glottal condition appears not to be valid.

(6) When electroglottograms are obtained simultaneously with other records on vocal fold vibration, such as stroboscopic imaging, ultra high speed films, photo-electric glottograms, or glottal airflow curves, a qualitative interpretation of the electroglottograms becomes possible.

# F. Ultrasound Glottography (Ultrasonoglottography)

Ultrasonic waves, that is, high frequency sound waves (1–10 MHz), can pass through various kinds of media, including body tissues. They are always reflected at the interface between two media which differ in specific acoustic impedance. The acoustic impedance is the numerical product of the density of the substance and the speed of the sound through it. The rate of energy reflection from the interface depends on the difference in acoustic impedance and on the angle of incidence relative to the interface. The difference in acoustic impedance between body tissues and the surrounding air is so large that transmission of ultrasound from the tissue to air is negligible. Making use of this fact, the opening and the closing of the glottis can be demonstrated.

Scientists at Chiba University developed a technique called "ultrasonoglottography" (Asano, 1968; Kitamura *et al.*, 1967; Kitamura *et al.*, 1969 a, b; Miura, 1969). In their technique, two transducers are placed on both sides of the neck and echoes from the vocal folds are recorded. The pulse beams transmitted through the glottis during the closed phase are also recorded simultaneously with the echo patterns (Fig. 4.10). Some other investigators have also attempted to use ultrasonic techniques in recording vocal fold vibration (Beach and Kelsey, 1969; Hamlet and Reid, 1972; Hamlet, 1973; Hamlet and Palmer, 1974; Holmer *et al.*, 1973; Holmer and Rundqvist, 1975; Minifie *et al.*, 1968).

The ultrasound glottogram can reflect the glottal condition during both the open and closed phases. Absolute values of the displacement of the vocal fold and the velocity of the movement are obtainable. However, a correct interpretation of the data obtained is not simple. The complicated shape of the vocal fold surface as the moving reflection interface and the up-and-down movement of the larynx relative to the transducers can be the major sources of artefacts.

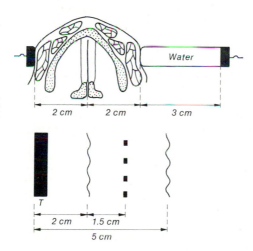

Fig. 4.10. Simultaneous recording of ultrasonoglottograms and closed phase (vertical dotted line) during vibratory cycle (Miura, 1969). *T* transmitted pulse

# References

## A. General

Hirano, M. (1975): Phonosurgery. Basic and clinical investigations. Otologia (Fukuoka) *21*, 239—442.

Hirano, M. (1976): Structure and vibratory behavior of the vocal folds. (U.S.—Japan Joint Seminar on Dynamic Aspects of Speech Production, December 7—10, Tokyo.)

Hirano, M., Koike, Y., Hirose, S., Morio, M. (1973): Structure of the vocal cord as a vibrator. J. Otolaryngol. Jpn. *76*, 1341—1348.

Hiroto, I. (1966): The mechanism of phonation. Its pathophysiological aspects. J. Otolaryngol. Jpn. *69*, 2097—2106.

## B. Stroboscopy

Baer, T. (1973): Measurement of vibration patterns of excised larynxes. QPR *110*, 169—175.

Beck, J., Schönhärl, E. (1954): Ein neues mikrophongesteuertes Lichtblitz-Stroboskop. HNO-Wegweiser *4*, 212—214.

Eigler, G., Podzuweit, G., Weiland, H. (1953): Ein neues mikrophongesteuertes Lichtblitz-Stroboskop zur Beobachtung von Stimmlippenschwingungen. Zschr. Laryng. Rhinol. *32*, 40.

Hirano, M., Nozoe, I., Shin, T., Maeyama, T. (1972): Vibration of the vocal cords recurrent laryngeal nerve palsy. A stroboscopic investigation. Pract. Otol. (Kyoto) *65*, 1037—1047.

Kirikae, I. (1943): Über den Bewegungsvorgang an den Stimmlippen und die Öffnungs- und Verschlußzeit der Stimmritze während der Phonation. J. Otolaryngol. Jpn. *49*, 236—262.

Mihashi, K. (1977): Investigations of phonatory function following vertical partial laryngectomy. Otologia (Fukuoka) *23*, 786—806.

Musehold, A. (1898): Stroboskopische und photographische Studien über die Stellung der Stimmlippen im Brust- und Falsett-Register. Arch. Laryngol. Rhinol. (Berlin) *7*, 1—21.

Oertel, M. (1825): Das Laryngo-Stroboskop und die laryngostroboskopische Untersuchung. Arch. Laryngol. Rhinol. (Berlin) *3*, 1—5.

Padovan, I. F., Christman, N. T., Hamlilton, L. (1973): Indirect microlaryngostroboscopy. Laryngoscope *83*, 2035—2041.

Panconcelli-Calzia, G. (1953): Das Synchron-Stroboskop nach Cremer. HNO *4*, 62.

Pantiukhin, V. P. (1954): Novaia model'stroboskopa. Vestn. Oto-rino-laryngol. *16*, 5.

Pascher, W., Homoth, R., Kruse, G. (1971): Verbesserte visuelle Diagnostik in der Laryngologie und Phoniatrie. HNO *19*, 373—375.

Saito, S. H. (1973): Microchirurgie stroboscopique du larynx. Rev. Laryng. *94*, 9—10.

Saito, S. (1977): Phonosurgery. Basic study on the mechanism of phonation and endolaryngeal microsurgery. Otologia (Fukuoka) *23*, 171—384.

Saito, S., Fukuda, H., Kitahara, S., Kokawa, N. (1978): Stroboscopic observation of vocal fold vibration with fiberoptics. Folia Phoniat. *30*, 241—244.

Schönhärl, E. (1960): Die Stroboskopie in der praktischen Laryngologie. Stuttgart: G. Thieme.

Seidner, W., Wendler, J., Halbedl, G. (1972): Mikrostroboskopie. Folia Phoniat. *24*, 81—85.

Shin, Y. (1976): Clinical and pathological investigations of sulcus vocalis. Otologia (Fukuoka) *22*, 819—835.

Timcke, R. (1956): Die Synchron-Stroboskopie von menschlichen „Stimmlippen bzw. ähnlichen Schallquellen und Messung der Öffnungszeit". Z. f. Laryng. Rhin. Otol. *35*, 331—335.

Vallancien, B. (1954): Le strobophone. Trans. Soc. de Laryngologie des Hopitaux de Paris.

von Leden, H. (1961): The electronic synchron-stroboscope. Ann. Otol. *70*, 881—893.

Winckel, F. (1954): Neuentwicklung eines Lichtblitz-Stroboskops für die Laryngologie. HNO-Wegweiser *4*, 210.

Yoshida, Y., Hirano, M., Nakajima, T. (1977): An improved model of laryngo-stroboscope. Otolaryngol. (Tokyo) *49*, 663—669.

Yoshida, Y., Hirano, M., Nakajima, T. (1979): A video-tape recording system for laryngo-stroboscopy. J. Jpn. Bronchoesophagol. Soc. *30*, 1—5.

## C. Ultra High Speed Photography

Bell Telephone Laboratories (1937): High speed motion pictures of the vocal cords. Bureau of Publication, Bell Telephone Laboratory, New York.

Dubovick, A. S. (1968): Photographic recording of high speed processes. London: Pergamon Press.

Dunker, E., Schlosshauer, B. (1958): Über Anspannung und Schwingungsform der Stimmlippen. Arch. Ohr. usw. Heilk. *173*, 497—500.

Fisher, H. B., Logemann, J. A. (1970): Objective evaluation of therapy for vocal nodules: A case report. J. Sp. Hear. Dis. *35*, 277—285.

Fransworth, D. W. (1940): High speed motion pictures of human vocal cords. Bell Telephone Laboratories.

Hayden, E. H., Koike, Y. (1972): A data processing scheme for frame-by-frame film analysis. Folia Phoniat. *24*, 169—181.

Hirano, M. (1970): Regulatory mechanism of voice in singing. Jpn. J. Logoped. Phoniat. *11*, 1—11.

Hirano, M. (1973): Vibration of the vocal cords in normal and pathological larynges (16-mm-Film).

Hirano, M., Kakita, Y., Kawasaki, H., Matsushita, H. (1977): Vocal cord vibration. Behavior of the layer-structured vibrator in normal and pathological conditions (16-mm-Film).

Hirano, M., Kawasaki, H., Matsushits, S., Toh, Y. (1978): Quantitative measurements of vocal fold vibration. An ultra high speed cinematographic investigation of normal subjects. J. Otolaryngol. Jpn. *81*, 820—826.

Hirano, M., Kawasaki, H., Matsushita, H., Yoshida, Y., Koike, Y. (1973): Mode of vocal cord vibration in recurrent laryngeal paralysis. J. Otolaryngol. Jpn. *76*, 721—728.

Hirano, M., Matsushita, H., Kawasaki, H., Yoshida, Y., Koike, Y. (1974): Vibration of the vocal cords with unilateral polyp. An ultra high speed cinematographic study. J. Otolaryngol. Jpn. *77*, 593—610.

Hirano, M., Matsushita, H., Kawasaki, H., Yoshida, Y., Yamaguchi, M., Ito, H. (1975): Application of computer to frame-by-frame analysis of vocal cord vibration. Pract. Otol. (Kyoto) *68*, 1289—1293.

Hirano, M., Miyahara, T., Miyagi, T., Kunitake, H., Nagashima, T., Matsushita, H., Maeyama, T., Sanui, N., Kawasaki, H., Nozoe, I., Hirose, H., Kiritani, S., Fujimura, O. (1971): Vocal regulation in singing. An experimental study in a professional singer. J. Otolaryngol. Jpn. *74*, 1189—1201.

Hirano, M., Yoshida, Y., Matsushita, H., Nakajima, T. (1974): An apparatus for ultra high speed cinematography of the vocal cords. Ann. Otol. *83*, 12—18.

Hiroto, I. (1966): Vibration of vocal cords, an ultra high speed cinematographic study (Motion picture).

Hiroto, I., Yoshida, Y., Nakajima, T. (1966): The investigation of the vocal cords vibration by the ultra high speed motion pictures, the photographing apparatus. Pract. Otol. (Kyoto) *59*, 47—55.

Hollien, H., Giard, G. T., Coleman, R. F. (1977): Vocal fold vibratory patterns of pulse resister phonation. Folia Phoniat. *29*, 200—205.

Isshiki, N., von Leden, H. (1963/1964): Laryngeal movements during cough. Studia Phonologia *3*, 1—6.

Kakita, Y., Hirano, M., Kawasaki, H., Matsushita, H. (1976): Schematical presentation of vibration of the vocal cord as a layer-structured vibrator. Normal larynges. J. Otolaryngol. Jpn. *79*, 1333—1340.

Kakita, Y., Hirano, M., Kawasaki, H., Matsushita, H. (1976): Schematical presentation of vibration of pathological vocal cords. J. Otolaryngol. Jpn. *79*, 1533—1548.

Kawasaki, H. (1976): Disorders in vibratory mode of some pathological vocal cords. A study with ultra high speed cinematography. Otologia (Fukuoka) *22*, 107—142.

Kobayashi, S. (1978): Glottal vibration after Hirano's reconstruction following hemilaryngectomy— An ultra high speed cinematographic investigation. Otologia (Fukuoka) *24*, 831—849.

Koike, Y., Hirano, M. (1973): Glottal-area time function and subglottal-pressure variation. J. Acoust. Soc. Amer. *54*, 1618—1627.

Le Cover, M., Rubin, H. J. (1960): Technique of high speed photography of the larynx. J. Biolog. Photogr. Assoc. *28*, 133—142.

Luchsinger, R., Pfister, K. (1959): Ergebnisse von Kehlkopfaufnahmen mit einer Zeitdehnerapparatur. Bull. Schweiz. Akad. Med. Wissensch. *15*, 164—177.

Matsushita, H. (1969): Vocal cord vibration of excised larynges. A study in the ultra high speed cinematography. Otologia (Fukuoka) *15*, 127—142.

Matsushita, H. (1975): The vibratory mode of the vocal fold in the excised larynx. Folia Phoniat. *27*, 7—18.

Moore, P., von Leden, H. (1958): Dynamic variations of the vibratory pattern in the normal larynx. Folia Phoniat. *10*, 205—238.

Moore, G. P., White, F. D., von Leden, H. (1962): Ultra high speed photography in laryngeal physiology. J. Sp. Hear. Dis. *27*, 165—171.

Ringel, R., Isshiki, N. (1964): Intra-oral voice recordings: on aid to laryngeal photography. Folia Phoniat. *16*, 19—28.

Rubin, H. J., Hirt, C. C. (1960): The falsetto a high speed cinematographic study. Laryngoscope *70*, 1305—1324.

Sonesson, B. (1960): On high speed filming of the human vocal folds. Communications from the Dept. of Anatomy, University of Lund, Sweden, No. 10.

Soron, H. I. (1967): High speed photography in speech research. J. Sp. Hear. Res. *10*, 768—776.

Tanabe, M. (1976): Effects of asymmetrical tension on the voice and vibratory pattern of the vocal cords. Pract. Otol. (Kyoto) *69*, 67—88.

Tanabe, M., Kitajima, K., Gould, W., Lambiase, A. (1975): Analysis of high speed motion picture of the vocal folds. Folia Phoniat. *27*, 77—87.

Teter, D. L., Newell, R. (1969): High speed photography of the larynx in a clinical setting. Ann. Otol. *78*, 1227—1233.

Timcke, R., von Leden, H., Moore, P. (1958): Laryngeal vibrations: measurements of the glottic wave. Part I. The normal vibratory cycle. Arch. Otolaryngol. *68*, 1—19.

Timcke, R., von Leden, H., Moore, P. (1959): Laryngeal vibrations: measurements of the glottic wave. Part II. Physiologic vibrations. Arch. Otolaryngol. *69*, 438—444.

Tsuiki, Y., Yamaguchi, T., Takakura, M. (1958): A study on the motion of the vocal cords during vocalization by means of high speed motion pictures. VII International Congress of Broncho-esophagology, Kyoto, Japan, p. 31.

von Leden, H. (1960): Laryngeal physiology cinematographic observation. J. Laryngol. *76*, 705—712.

von Leden, H., Isshiki, N. (1965): An analysis of cough at the level of the larynx. Arch. Otolaryngol. *81*, 616—625.

von Leden, H., Le Cover, M., Ringel, R. L., Isshiki, N. (1966): Improvements in laryngeal cinematography. Arch. Otolaryngol. *83*, 482—487.

von Leden, H., Moore, P. (1961): Vibratory pattern of the vocal cords in unilateral laryngeal paralysis. Acta Otolaryngol. *53*, 493—506.

von Leden, H., Moore, P., Timcke, R. (1960): Laryngeal vibrations: Measurements of the glottic wave. Part III. The pathologic larynx. Arch. Otolaryngol. *71*, 16—35.

Yoshida, Y. (1969): An investigation of vocal cord vibration by means of ultra high speed photography. J. Otolaryngol. Jpn. *72*, 1232—1250.

Yoshida, Y., Hirano, M., Matsushita, H., Nakajima, T. (1972): A new apparatus for ultra high speed cinematography of vibrating vocal cords (Ultra High Laryngocine Model Ku-II). J. Otolaryngol. Jpn. *75*, 1256—1262.

## D. Photo-Electric Glottography

Coleman, R. F., Wendal, R. W. (1968): On the validity of laryngeal photosensor monitoring. J. Acoust. Soc. Amer. *44*, 1733—1735.

Fant, G., Sonesson, B. (1962): Indirect studies of glottal cycles by synchronous inverse filtering and photoelectrical glottography. Speech Transmission Lab. Quart. Prog. Status Rep., Royal Inst. Technol. (Stockholm) *4*, 1—3.

Frøkjaer-Jensen, B. (1967): A photo-electric glottograph. Annual Report of the Institute of Phonetics of Univ. Copenhagen *2*, 5—19.

Kitzing, P., Sonesson, B. (1974): A photoglottographical study of the female vocal folds during phonation. Folia Phoniat. *26*, 138—149.

Lisker, L., Abramson, A. S., Cooper, F. S., Schvey, M. H. (1969): Transillumination of the larynx in running speech. J. Acoust. Soc. Amer. *45*, 1544—1546.

Malécot, A., Peebles, K. (1965): An optical device for recording glottal adduction-abduction during normal speech. Zphon *18*, 545—550.

Ohara, J. (1966): An new photo-electric glottograph. Working Papers in Phonetics, Univ. of California (Los Angeles) *4*, 40—52.

Sawashima, M. (1968): Movements of the larynx in articulation of Japanese consonants. Annual Bulletin (Research Institute of Logopedics and Phoniatrics, Univ. Tokyo), no. 2, 11—20.

Slis, J. H., Damsté, P. H. (1967): Transillumination of the glottis during voiced and voiceless consonants. IPO Annual Progress Report no. 2, 103—109, Eindhoven, Holland.

Sonesson, B. (1959): A method for studying the vibratory movements of the vocal cords. A preliminary report. J. Laryngol. *73*, 732—737.

Sonesson, B. (1960): On the anatomy and vibratory pattern of the human vocal folds. With special reference to a photoelectrical method for studying the vibratory movements. Acta Otolaryngol. Suppl. *156*, 1—80.

## E. Electroglottography

Chevrie-Muller, C. (1962): Etude de l'électroglottogramme et du phonogramme en période de "mue vocale". Ann. Otolaryngol. (Paris) *79*, 1035—1044.

Chevrie-Muller, C. (1964): Etude de fonctionnement laryngé chez les bègues par la méthode glottografique. Rev. Laryngol. (Bordeaux) *85*, 763—774.

Chevrie-Muller, C. (1967): Contribution à l'étude des traces glottographiques chez l'adulte normal. Rev. Laryngol. (Bordeaux) *88*, 227—243.

Fabre, M. P. (1957): Un procédé électrique percutané d'inscription de l'accolement glottique au cours de la phonation: Glottographie de haute fréquence. Premiers résultats. Bull. Acad. nat. Méd. *141*, 66—69.

Fabre, M. P. (1958): Etude comparée des glottogrammes et des phonogrammes de la voix humaine. Ann. Otolaryngol. (Paris) *75*, 767—775.

Fabre, M. P. (1961): Glottographie respiratoire: Appareillage et premiers résultats. C. R. Acad. Sci. (Paris) *252*, 1386—1388.

Fabre, M. P. (1961): Glottographie respiratoire. Ann. Otolaryngol. (Paris) *78*, 814—824.

Fant, G., Ondráčková, J., Lindqvist, J., Sonesson, B. (1966): Electrical glottography. STL-QPSR 4/1966, 15—21.

Fischer-Jørgensen, E., Frøkjaer-Jensen, B., Rischel, J. (1966): Preliminary experiments with the Fabre glottograph. Annual Report of the Institute of Phonetics of Univ. Copenhagen *1*, 22—29.

Fourcin, A. J. (1974): Laryngographic examination of vocal fold vibration. In: An International Symposium of Ventilatory and Phonatory Control System, p. 315. London: Oxford University Press.

Fourcin, A. J. (1979): Laryngographic Assessment of Phonatory Function (NIH Conference on the Assessment of Vocal Pathology).

Fourcin, A. J., Abberton, E. (1971): First applications of a new laryngograph. Med. Biol. Illustr. *21*, 172—182.

Fourcin, A. J., Norgate, M. (1965): Measurement of the transglottal impedance. Progress Report, Phon. Lab., Univ. College, London.

Fourcin, A. J., West, J. E. (1968): Larynx movement detector, Extr. Progress Report, Phon. Lab., Univ. College, London.

Frøkjaer-Jensen, B. (1968): Comparison between a Fabre glottograph and a photo-electric glottograph. Annual Report of the Institute of Phonetics of Univ. Copenhagen *3*, 9—16.

Frøkjaer-Jensen, B., Thorvaldsen, P. (1968): Construction of a Fabre glottograph. Annual Report of the Institute of Phonetics of Univ. Copenhagen *3*, 1—8.

Gougerot, L., Grémy, F., Marstal, N. (1960): Glottographie à large bande passante. Application à l'étude de la voix de fausset. J. Physiol. *52*, 823—832.

Grémy, F. (1963): Etude du glottogramme chez l'enfant sourd en cours de rééducation vocale. Ann. Otolaryngol. (Paris) *80*, 803—815.

Holm, C. (1969): Das Verhalten von Vokalen und Konsonanten im phono- und elektroglottographischen Bild. Arch. Ohr. usw. Heilk. *194*, 258—260.

Holm, C. (1970): Erste Ergebnisse einer Elektroglottographie im Kindesalter. Arch. Ohr. usw. Heilk. *196*, 359—363.

Holm, C. (1971): L'évolution de la phonation de la première enfance à la puberté: une étude électroglottographique. J. Franc. ORL *20*, 437—440.

Jentzsch, H., Sasama, R., Unger, E. (1978): Elektroglottographische Untersuchungen zur Problematik des Stimmeinsatzes bei zusammenhängendem Sprechen. Folia Phoniat. *30*, 59—66.

Kitzing, P. (1977): Methode zur kombinierten photo- und elektroglottographischen Registrierung von Stimmlippenschwingungen. Folia Phoniat. 29, 249—260.

Köster, J. P., Smith, S. V. (1970): Zur Interpretation elektrischer und photoelektrischer Glottogramme. Folia Phoniat. 22, 92—99.

Lebrun, Y. (1971): On the so-called "Dissociations" between electroglottogram and phonogram. Folia Phoniat. 23, 225—227.

Lecluse, F. L. E. (1976): Laboratory investigations in electroglottography. Proc. 16th Int. Congr. Log. Phon., 1974. Basel: Karger.

Lecluse, F. L. E. (1977): Quantitative measurements in electroglottography. 17th Int. Congr. Log. Phon., Copenhagen (in press).

Lecluse, F. L. E. (1977): Elektroglottographie. Utrecht: Drukkerijelinkwijk B.V.

Lecluse, F. L. E., Brocaar, M. P., Verschuure, J. (1975): The electroglottography and its relation to glottal activity. Folia Phoniat. 27, 215—224.

Loebell, E. (1968): Über den klinischen Wert der Elektroglottographie. Arch. Ohr. usw. Heilk. 191, 760—764.

Loebell, E. (1970): Neue Ergebnisse der Elektroglottographie (EGG), IX. Welt-HNO-Kongreß-Verhandlungen, Mexico City.

Neil, W. F., Wechsler, E., Robinson, J. M. P. (1977): Electrolaryngography in laryngeal disorders. Clin. Otolaryngol. 2, 33—40.

Ondráčková, J. (1972): Vocal-chord activity. Its dynamics and role in speech production. Folia Phoniat. 24, 405—419.

Pedersen, M. F. (1977): Electroglottography compared with synchronized stroboscopy in normal person. Folia Phoniat. 29, 191—199.

Reinsch, M., Gobsch, H. (1972): Zur quantitativen Auswertung elektroglottographischer Kurven bei Normalpersonen. Folia Phoniat. 24, 1—6.

Striglioni, L. (1963): Contribution à l'étude de la physiologie du larynx en voix parlée. Apport de l'électroglottographie, Thesis, Marseille.

Vallancien, B., Faulhaber, J. (1967): What to think of glottography. Folia Phoniat. 19, 39—44.

Vallancien, B., Gautheron, P. L., Guisez, D., Paley, B. (1971): Comparison des singnaux microphoniques, diaphonographiques et glottographiques, avec application au laryngographe. Folia Phoniat. 23, 371—380.

van Michel, C. L. (1964): Etude par la méthode électroglottographique, des comportements glottiques de type phonatoire en dehors de toute émission sonore. Rev. Laryngol. 7—8, 469—475.

van Michel, C. L. (1966): Mouvements glottiques phonatoires sans émission sonore, Etude électroglottographique. Folia Phoniat. 18, 1—18.

van Michel, C. L. (1967): Morphologie de la courbe glottographique dans certains troubles fonctionnels du larynx. Folia Phoniat. 19, 192—202.

van Michel, C. L., Pfister, K. A., Luchsinger, R. (1970): Electroglottographie et cinématographie laryngée ultrarapide. Folia Phoniat. 22, 81—99.

van Michel, C. L., Raskin, L. (1969): L'électroglottomètre Mark 4, son principe, ses possibilités. Folia Phoniat. 21, 145—157.

## F. Ultrasound Glottography

Asano, H. (1968): Application of the ultrasonic pulse-method on the larynx. J. Otolaryngol. Jpn. 71, 895—916.

Beach, J. L., Kelsey, C. A. (1969): Ultrasonic doppler monitoring of vocal fold velocity and displacement. J. Acoust. Soc. Amer. 46, 1045—1047.

Hamlet, S. L. (1972): Vocal fold articulatory activity during whispered sibilants. Arch. Otolaryngol. 95, 211—213.

Hamlet, S. L. (1973): Vocal compensation: an ultrasonic study of vocal fold vibration in normal and nasal vowels. Cleft Palate J. 10, 367—385.

Hamlet, S. L., Palmer, J. M. (1974): An investigation of laryngeal trills using the transmission of ultrasound through the larynx. Folia Phoniat. 26, 362—378.

Hamlet, S. L., Reid, J. M. (1972): Transmission of ultrasound through the larynx as a means of determining vocal fold activity. IEEE Trans. Biomed. Eng. 19, 34—37.

Hertz, C. H., Lindström, K., Sonesson, B. (1970): Ultrasonic recording of the vibrating vocal folds. Acta Otolaryng. *69,* 223—230.

Holmer, N. G., Kitzing, P., Lindström, K. (1973): Echo glottography. Ultrasonic recording of vocal fold vibrations in preparations of human larynges. Acta Otolaryng. *75,* 454—463.

Holmer, N. G., Rundqvist, H. E. (1975): Ultrasonic registration of the fundamental frequency of a voice during normal speech. J. Acoust. Soc. Amer. *58,* 1073—1077.

Kaneko, T., Kobayashi, N., Asano, H., Miura, T., Naito, J., Hayasaki, K., Kitamura, T. (1974): L'ultra-sonoglottographie. Ann. Otolaryng. (Paris) *7—8,* 403—410.

Kaneko, T., Kobayashi, N., Tachibana, M., Naito, J., Hayasaki, K., Uchida, T., Yoshioka, T., Suzuki, H. (1976): L'ultrasonoglottographie; l'aire neutre glottique et la vibration de la corde vocale. Rev. de Laryngol. *97,* 9—10.

Kitamura, T., Kaneko, T., Asano, H. (1964): Ultrasonic diagnosis of the laryngeal diseases. Jpn. Med. Ultrason. *2,* 14—15.

Kitamura, T., Kaneko, T., Asano, H., Miura, T. (1967): Ultrasonoglottography. A preliminary report. Jpn. Med. Ultrason. *5,* 40—41.

Kitamura, T., Kaneko, T., Asano, H., Miura, T. (1969a): L'ultrasonoglottographie. Revue de Laryngol. *3—4,* 190—195.

Kitamura, T., Kaneko, T., Asano, H., Miura, T. (1969b): Ultrasonic diagnosis in otorhinolaryngology. Eye, Ear, Nose and Throat Monthly *48,* 121—131.

Minifie, F. D., Kelsey, C. A., Hixon, T. J. (1968): Measurement of vocal fold motion using an ultrasonic doppler velocity monitor. JASA *43,* 1165—1169.

Miura, T. (1969): Mode of vocal card vibration. A study with ultrasonoglottography. J. Otolaryngol. Jpn. *72,* 985—1002.

# 5 Acoustic Analysis of the Voice Signal

Acoustic analysis of the voice signal may be one of the most attractive methods for assessing phonatory function or laryngeal pathology because it is non-invasive and provides objective and quantitative data. On the other hand, for well-trained laryngologists, phoniatricians or speech pathologists listening to the patient's voice can provide a fairly accurate guide to the possible causes of the patient's voice disorder. These facts strongly support the assertion that the technique of acoustic analysis has a promising future as a diagnostic tool in the management of voice disorders. Many acoustic parameters, derived by various methods, have been reported to be useful in differentiating between the pathological voice and the normal voice. All the previous reports are, however, preliminary studies. Further extensive basic and clinical research is required in order to obtain some algorithm for diagnostic purposes.

In this chapter, a review of previous studies is made so as to summarize the concept of acoustic analysis.

## A. Signal Source for Acoustic Analysis

### 1. Oral-Output Signal

The most readily available signal for acoustic analysis is the sound pressure waveform emanating from the mouth (oral-output signal). It can be tape-recorded or fed into analytical systems via a microphone placed in front of the subject's mouth. The usefulness of the signal obtained in this manner, however, is limited. The acoustic features of the oral-output signal are determined not only by the glottal sound but also by the transmission characteristics of the vocal tract and lip radiation characteristics (Fig. 5.1). In assessing vocal function, the glottal sound must be examined.

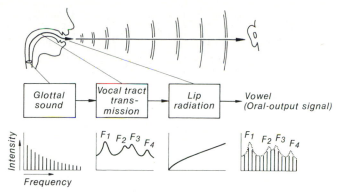

Fig. 5.1. Determinants of the spectrum of a vowel (oral-output signal)

## 2. Pre-Tracheal or Pre-Laryngeal Vibration

In order to reduce the effects of the vocal tract a pre-tracheal (or pre-laryngeal) contact microphone is sometimes used. This is a simple technique. However, it is unknown to what extent the effects of the supraglottic structures are reduced. Furthermore, information derived from pre-tracheal contact signals is limited by the low-pass filtering effect of the intervening structures.

## 3. Glottal Sound Wave Derived by Inverse Filtering Based on a Physical Model

The idea of inverse filtering is to obtain the glottal sound, or glottal volume velocity waveform, by eliminating the contribution from the vocal tract transmission and lip radiation from the oral-output signal. The technique is theoretically based on the vowel production model as a linear physical system (Fant, 1960; Flanagan, 1972). Use of the digital computer has facilitated technical progress. However, precise determination of the formant frequencies and bandwidths for each oral-output signal is tedious. In addition, an FM tape-recorder is required because any low frequency phase distortion which is inherent in regular tape-recorders interferes with accurate approximation of the glottal sound source.

## 4. Residue Wave Derived by the Inverse Filtering Based on Linear Prediction

This filtering technique is theoretically based on a mathematical model called the linear prediction model of speech production (Atal and Hanauer, 1971; Makhoul, 1975; Markel and Gray, 1976). The inverse filter in this case is equivalent to a combination of the inverse characteristics of the lip radiation, vocal tract and glottal shaping spectral contribution to the oral-output signal, *i.e.* speech signal. The residue signal which is obtained by filtering the speech signal with this filter is an estimate of a periodic source signal which is theoretically an impulse train. Since it is

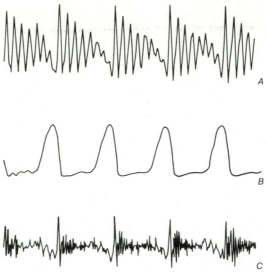

Fig. 5.2. Comparison of speech, glottal sound and residue signals for /a/. The glottal sound signal is closely correlated with the physiological glottal volume velocity waveform (Davis, 1976). *A* Original speech waveform, *B* Glottal sound signal derived from speech waveform with a physical inverse filtering, *C* Residue signal derived from speech waveform with a linear prediction inverse filtering

a hypothetical input signal, it is not directly related to any physically observable signal. It can be, however, obtained automatically and more easily than the glottal sound waveform obtained with the physical inverse filtering technique. Fig. 5.2 compares the speech, glottal sound and residue signals.

## 5. Glottal Sound Wave Derived by a Reflectionless Tube (Sondhi's Tube)

This technique employs a long reflectionless tube (Fig. 5.3) which is considered to act as a pseudo-infinite termination of the vocal tract. When a subject produces a neutral vowel into the tube, a microphone within the tube picks up the glottal source waveform, because the reflectionless termination of the tube significantly reduces the resonant characteristics of the vocal tract. Each subject requires a different tube which matches his/her vocal tract. This method was originally

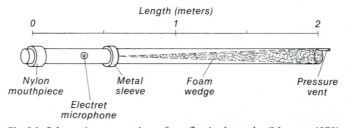

Fig. 5.3. Schematic presentation of a reflectionless tube (Monsen, 1979)

described by Sondhi (1975). Under ideal conditions, it should be an easy, simple and quick means of obtaining the glottal source waveform. Recordings reported previously, however, were not very satisfactory.

# B. Sample for Acoustic Analysis

## 1. Steady Portion of Sustained Vowel

Since it is easier to estimate the effects of vocal tract transmission and lip radiation, the steady portion of a sustained vowel has been most frequently used as a sample for acoustic analysis. The steady portion of a sustained vowel should be the standard sample for acoustic analysis.

## 2. Transitional Parts of Phonation

Many pathological conditions are more apparent during the transitional phases of phonation, including the onset and the termination of phonation and hence of speech. There is no standard procedure for selecting such samples. Adequate selection of such samples depends largely on the clinician's experience. In this connection, further extensive clinical and basic research is also required.

# C. Acoustic Parameters for the Assessment of Vocal Function

## 1. General Description

The acoustic parameters relevant for the assessment of vocal function are those which demonstrate one or more of the following aspects of the voice signal.

*(1) Fundamental Frequency or Fundamental Period*
    a) The mean of a given phonation
    b) The possible range of a given subject (frequency range of phonation)
    c) Fluctuation in a given phonation
        (1) Extent of the fluctuation
        (2) Periodicity of the fluctuation

*(2) Intensity, Sound Pressure or Amplitude of the Acoustic Waveform*
    a) The mean of a given phonation
    b) The possible range of a given subject (intensity range of phonation)
    c) Fluctuation in a given phonation
        (1) Extent of the fluctuation
        (2) Periodicity of the fluctuation

*(3) The Amount of or Richness in Spectral Harmonics*
    a) The mean of a given phonation
    b) Fluctuation in a given phonation
        (1) Extent of the fluctuation
        (2) Periodicity of the fluctuation

*(4) Amount of Noise (Turbulent Air Noise)*
    a) The mean of a given phonation
    b) Fluctuation in a given phonation
        (1) Extent of the fluctuation
        (2) Periodicity of the fluctuation

## 2. Parameters Related to Fundamental Frequency

Various statistics can be derived from a series of values of successive fundamental periods (Fig. 5.4).

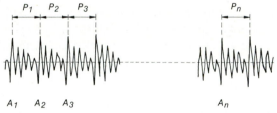

Fig. 5.4. Series of fundamental periods *(P$_1$, P$_2$, P$_3$, ... P$_n$)* and amplitudes *(A$_1$, A$_2$, A$_3$, ... A$_n$)*

*(1) Standard Statistics*

    a) Mean ($\bar{P}$)

$$\bar{P} = \frac{1}{n} \sum_{i=1}^{n} P_1$$

    b) Standard deviation ($\sigma$)

$$\sigma = \sqrt{\frac{1}{n} \sum_{i=1}^{n} (P_1 - \bar{P})^2}$$

    c) Coefficient of variation (v)

$$v = \frac{\sigma}{\bar{P}}$$

*(2) Parameters Specially Proposed*

    a) "Pitch perturbation" (Lieberman, 1963)
    "Pitch perturbation ($\Delta$P)" is defined as the value obtained by subtracting the duration of a period (P$_i$) from the period immediately preceeding it (P$_{i-1}$).

$$\Delta P = P_{i-1} - P_i$$

b) "Pitch perturbation factor" (Lieberman, 1963)

"Pitch perturbation factor (PPF)" is defined as the relative frequency of pitch perturbation of 0.5 msec or greater occurring in a given phonatory sample.

$$PPF = \frac{\text{frequency of } \Delta P \text{ of 0.5 msec or greater}}{\text{total number of } \Delta P \text{ in a given sample}}$$

c) "Relative average perturbation" (Koike, 1973)

Koike observed that steady phonation normally shows slow and relatively smooth changes in fundamental period, and he attempted to measure rapid perturbations from a smoothened trend line. He also normalized the degree of perturbation by dividing it by the average fundamental period. Thus, he defined the relative average perturbation (RAP) as:

$$RAP = \frac{\dfrac{1}{n-2} \displaystyle\sum_{i=2}^{n-1} \left| \dfrac{P_{i-1} + P_i + P_{i+1}}{3} - P_i \right|}{\dfrac{1}{n} \displaystyle\sum_{i=1}^{n} P_1}$$

Similar ideas were presented by Takahashi and Koike (1975) and Davis (1976).

### (3) Correlogram

A graphic presentation of the serial correlation coefficients for the time series of a given value is called a correlogram. The serial correlation coefficient for a given lag K ($r_k$) is defined by the following formula:

$$r_k = \frac{1}{N-k} \sum_{i=1}^{N-k} x_1 \cdot x_{1+k} - \bar{x}_1 \bar{x}_2 \bigg/ s_1 s_2,$$

where

$$\bar{x}_1 = \sum_{i=1}^{N-k} x_1 \bigg/ (N-k), \quad \bar{x}_2 = \sum_{i=k+1}^{N} x_1 \bigg/ (N-k),$$

$$s_1^2 = \sum_{i=1}^{N-k} \frac{(x_1 - \bar{x}_1)^2}{N-k}, \quad s_2^2 = \sum_{i=k+1}^{N} \frac{(x_1 - \bar{x}_2)^2}{N-k}.$$

Lieberman (1963) first reported that the "pitch perturbation factor" was greater for the pathological voice than for the normal voice. Since then, parameters which demonstrate cycle-to-cycle fluctuations of fundamental period have been investigated by some clinicians and voice scientists (Davis, 1976; Kitajima et al., 1975; Koike, 1973; Takahashi and Koike, 1975; Wendahl, 1963 and 1966; Hiki et al., 1976; Iwata and von Leden, 1970; Iwata, 1972).

## 3. Parameters Related to Vocal Intensity

Statistics identical to those for fundamental frequency as described in the previous section can be derived from a series of values of the wave amplitude of successive periods. It should be kept in mind that the maximum amplitude of a given waveform is not always proportional to the sound pressure. With regard to the glottic volume velocity waveform, for example, the sound pressure is a function not only of the maximum amplitude but also of some other factors such as the open quotient.

Koike (1969) first paid attention to the cycle-to-cycle amplitude variations in pathological voices and showed differences between normal and pathological voices (Fig. 5.5). Davis (1976) and Hiki *et al.* (1976) adopted acoustic parameters related to amplitude fluctuation in their investigations of pathological voices.

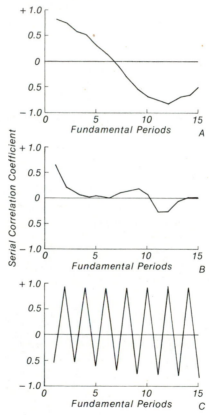

Fig. 5.5. Correlograms of the amplitude values obtained from a normal subject *(A)*, a patient with unilateral laryngeal paralysis *(B)*, and a patient with laryngeal cancer *(C)*. (Koike, 1969)

## 4. Spectral Harmonics and Noise

Quantification of spectral harmonics and noise in voice signals is not an easy task. The following attempts have been made by several investigators.

## a) Sound Spectrography

On the basis of sound spectrographic analysis of hoarse voices, Yanagihara (1967 a, b) proposed a classification of hoarseness into four types. He also related these types to the vibratory pattern of the vocal folds and the mean airflow rate.

Type I: The regular harmonic components are mixed with the noise component chiefly in the formant region of the vowels.

Type II: The noise components in the second formants of /e/ and /i/ predominate over the harmonic components, and slight additional noise components appear in the high frequency region above 3000 Hz in the vowels /e/ and /i/.

Type III: The second formants of /e/ and /i/ are totally replaced by noise components, and the additional noise components above 3000 Hz further intensify their energy and expand their range.

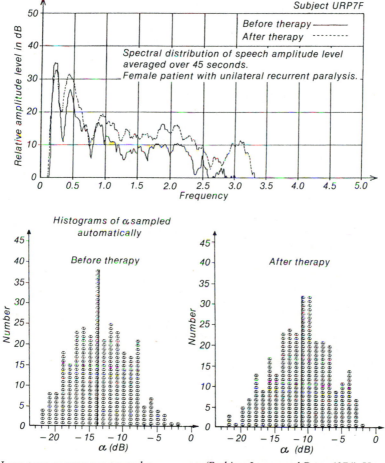

Fig. 5.6. Long-term-average-spectra and α-parameter (Frøkjaer-Jensen and Prytz, 1976). Upper graph: LTAS-analysis of a patient suffering from unilateral paralysis before and after treatment. Lower graphs: Distribution of the amplitude above 1000 Hz relative to the amplitude below 1000 Hz, sampled automatically 25 times per second

Type IV: The second formants of /a/, /e/ and /i/ are replaced by noise components, and even the first formants of all vowels often lose their periodic components which are supplemented by noise components. In addition, more intensive high frequency noise components are present.

## b) Long-Time-Average-Spectra (LTAS, Frøkjaer-Jensen and Prytz, 1976)

Using a 400 channel Real Time Narrow Band Analyzer and a CRT display unit, spectral distribution of speech amplitude level averaged over 45 sec is displayed. Changes in voice quality by therapy are demonstrated (Fig. 5.6).

## c) α-parameter (Frøkjaer-Jensen and Prytz, 1976)

The α-parameter is defined as:

$$\alpha = \frac{\text{amplitude level above 1000 Hz}}{\text{amplitude level below 1000 Hz}}$$

# 5. Multidimensional Approach

Since any single acoustic parameter is not sufficient to demonstrate the entire spectrum of vocal function or of laryngeal pathologies, multidimensional analysis using multiple acoustic parameters has been attempted by some investigators.

## a) Application of Residue Signals

Davis (1976) derived the following six acoustic parameters from residue signals.
  (1) Pitch perturbation quotient (PPQ)

$$PPQ = \frac{\frac{1}{n-(k-1)} \sum_{i=1}^{n-(k-1)} \left| \frac{1}{k} \sum_{j=1}^{k} P(i+j-1) - P(i+m) \right|}{\left| \frac{1}{n} \sum_{i=1}^{n} P(i) \right|}$$

Where k is the length of moving average (an odd integer greater than one) and $m = (k+1)/2$.
  (2) Amplitude perturbation quotient (APQ)
    APQ is analogous to PPQ.
  (3) Pitch amplitude (PA)
    PA is defined as the value of pitch period peak in the residue signal autocorrelation sequence for a vowel sound.
  (4) Coefficient of excess (EX)
    Koike and Markel (1975) noticed that a visual judgment of the signal-to-noise ratio of the residue signal is qualitatively correlated with the degree of severity

of the pathological state in most cases. The "signal" here is the sequence of spikes spaced at pitch period intervals and the "noise" is the randomly appearing energy between the spikes. Davis (1976) adopted a statistical measure called the coefficient of excess (Cramer, 1958) in an attempt to quantify the visual differences. EX is defined as the ratio of the fouth moment of the signal to the square of the second moment of the signal.

(5) Spectral flatness of the inverse filter spectrum (SFF)

This is equivalent to the spectral slope of the glottal waveform represented in dB/oct, and is negative in value. As the noise level increases, the SFF increases.

(6) Spectral flatness of the residue signal spectrum (SFR)

This represents the spectral slope of the residue signal measured in dB/oct. Davis (1976) suggested that the SFR might be regarded as a measure of the masking of the fundamental frequency harmonic amplitudes by noise. As noise level increases, the SFR increases.

Using these six parameters, Davis made multidimensional analysis aiming at differentiation of pathological voices from normal voices. The detection probability was 95.2 per cent in a closed test and 67.4 per cent in an open test.


## b) Application of Glottal Waveform

Hiki, Hirano and their co-workers reported a series of investigations of acoustic analysis of pathological voices (Hiki *et al.,* 1976; Hirano, 1975; Hirano *et al.,* 1976; Hirano *et al.,* 1977 a, b; Hirano *et al.,* 1979; Kakita *et al.,* 1977 a, b). From the glottal sound waveform obtained with an inverse filtering technique, they derived the following 14 acoustic parameters:

(1) Amplitude of second crest of the autocorrelation function (Po).
(2) Width of second crest of the autocorrelation function (Wl).
(3) Amplitude of first trough of the autocorrelation function (MP).
(4) Standard deviation of fundamental period (PDEV).
(5) Standard deviation of peak amplitude (ADEV).
(6) Period of fluctuation of the correlogram of fundamental period (PPER).
(7) Period of fluctuation of the correlogram of peak amplitude (APER).
(8) Correlation coefficient between adjacent fundamental periods (Pl).
(9) Correlation coefficient between fundamental periods separated by ten intervals (P10).
(10) Rate of declination of the correlogram of fundamental period (PINC).
(11) Correlation coefficient between adjacent peak amplitude (Al).
(12) Correlation coefficient between peak amplitudes separated by ten intervals (A10).
(13) Rate of declination of the correlogram of peak amplitude (AINC).
(14) Rate of declination of spectral envelope (SPINC).

They related these acoustic parameters to other factors which relate to phonatory function, including vibratory pattern of the vocal folds, physical properties of the vocal folds, aerodynamic measures and psycho-acoustic parameters of the voice. They finally made canonical analysis using the 14 acoustic parameters with

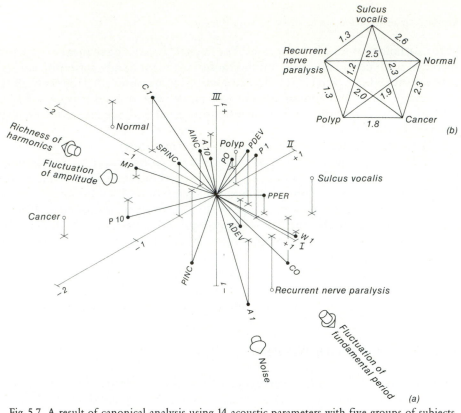

Fig. 5.7. A result of canonical analysis using 14 acoustic parameters with five groups of subjects (Kakita *et al.*, 1977b)

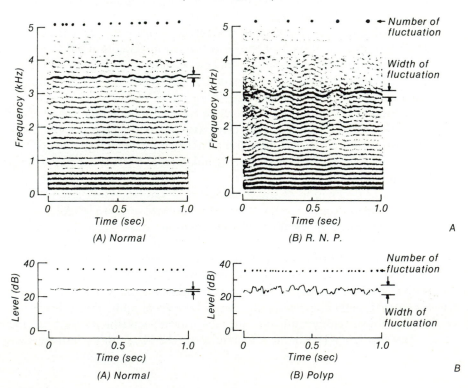

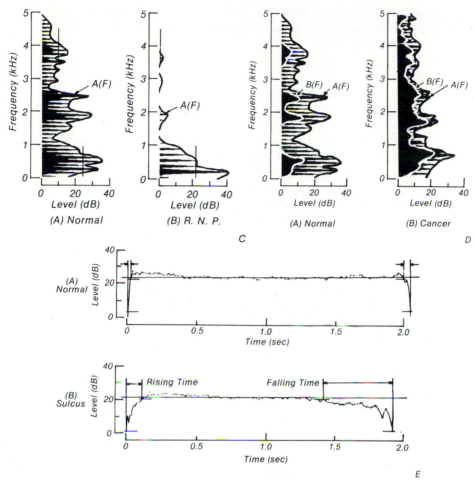

Fig. 5.8. Acoustic parameters obtained from sound spectrograms (Imaizumi *et al.*, 1980). *A* Size and speed of fundamental frequency fluctuation. *B* Size and speed of overall amplitude fluctuation. *C* Richness of high frequency harmonics demonstrated by the ratio of the mean level of the frequency range between 3.5 to 4.5 KHz to that below 1 KHz. *D* Relative noise level demonstrated by the difference between the two envelopes, A(F) and B(F). *A(F)* Envelope obtained by connecting the peaks of the harmonics. *B(F)* Envelope obtained by connecting the troughs of the section display. *E* Rising time and falling time. *R.N.P.* Recurrent laryngeal nerve paralysis

five groups of subjects: normal, carcinoma, recurrent laryngeal nerve paralysis, polyp and sulcus vocalis. The results revealed that 70–80% of the subjects in each group were separated from other groups (Fig. 5.7).

## c) Application of Sound Spectrogram

The inverse filtering technique and many other methods of acoustic analysis require a computer system, which is expensive and, therefore, not available in most voice clinics. A sound spectrograph is more readily available than a computer system in many clinics. Imaizumi *et al.* (1980) investigated the possibility of utilizing a sound spectrograph for a multidimensional analysis of pathological voices. They measured the following nine acoustic parameters from sound spectrograms of sustained vowels (Fig. 5.8):

(1) Size of fundamental frequency fluctuation. This is measured on a narrow-filter standard pattern. The size of fluctuation is represented by the ratio of the peak-to-peak value ($\Delta F_0$) and the mean fundamental frequency ($\overline{F}_0$).

(2) Speed of fundamental frequency fluctuation. This is shown by the number of the positive peaks within one second.

(3) Size of overall amplitude fluctuation. This is measured on an amplitude display by determining the peak-to-peak value.

(4) Speed of overall amplitude fluctuation. This is defined as the number of the positive peaks within one second on an amplitude display.

(5) Richness of high frequency harmonics. A section display is used in quantifying this parameter. They adopted a ratio of the mean level of the frequency range between 3.5 to 4.5 KHz to that below 1 KHz.

(6) Relative noise level. This is estimated on a section display. They obtained two envelopes: one by connecting the peaks of the harmonics and the other by connecting the troughs of the section display. They thought that the latter could be regarded as a measure of the noise level except for voices of low fundamental frequencies. The difference between the two envelopes was adopted as the parameter which indicates the relative noise level. They measured the relative noise level in two frequency ranges: the range of the first formant and that of the second formant.

(7) Rising time and falling time. These two parameters are measured on an amplitude display. The rising time was defined as the time required for the increase in the overall amplitude from the value of 10% of the steady level to 90%. The falling time was defined as the time span required for the decrease from 90% to 10% of the steady level.

# References

Atal, B. S., Hanauer, S. L. (1971): Speech analysis and synthesis by linear prediction of the speech wave. J. Acoust. Soc. Amer. *50*, 637–655.

Beckett, R. L. (1969): Pitch perturbation as a function of subjective vocal construction. Folia Phoniat. *21*, 416–425.

Bowler, N. W. (1964): A fundamental frequency analysis of harsh vocal quality. Speech Monogr. *31*, 128–134.

Buch, N. H., Frøkjaer-Jensen, B. (1972): Some remarks on acoustic parameters in speech disorders. Annual Report of the Institute of Phonetics Univ. Copenhagen 6, 245–258.

Burger, D., van den Verg, J. W. (1962): Experimental askiness (hoarseness). Pract. ORL *24*, 192.

Coleman, R. F. (1971): Effect of waveform changes upon roughness perception. Folia Phoniat. *23*, 314–322.

Cooper, M. (1974): Spectrographic analysis of fundamental frequency and hoarseness before and after vocal rehabilitation. J. Sp. Hear. Dis. *39*, 286–297.

Cramer, H. (1958): Mathematical Methods of Statistics. Princeton: Princeton University Press.

Davis, S. B. (1976): Computer evaluation of laryngeal pathology based on inverse filtering of speech. Ph. D. Dissertation, University of California, Santa Barbara. Also SCRL Monograph *13*, Speech Communications Research Laboratory, Inc., Santa Barbara.

Davis, S. (1979): NIH Conference on the Assessment of Vocal Pathology.

Fant, C. G. M. (1960): Acoustic Theory of Speech Production. 's Gravenhage: Mouton and Co.

Flanagan, J. L. (1958): Some properties of the glottal sound source. J. Sp. Hear. Res. *1*, 99—116.

Flanagan, J. L. (1972): Speech Analysis, Synthesis and Perception. Berlin-Heidelberg-New York: Springer.

Fritzell, B., Hammarberg, B. (1977): Cinical applications of acoustic voice analysis. Background and perceptual factors. I.A.L.P. Congress Proc. *1*, 477—487.

Frøkjaer-Jensen, B., Prytz, S. (1976): Registration of voice quality. Bruel and Kjar Technical Review No. 3, 3—17.

Gauffin, J., Sundberg, J. (1977): Clinical applications of acoustic voice analysis. Acoustical analysis, results and discussion. I.A.L.P. Congress Proc. *1*, 489—502.

Hecker, M. H. I., Kreul, E. J. (1971): Description of the speech of patients with cancer of the vocal folds. Part I: Measurements of fundamental frequency. J. Acoust. Soc. Amer. *49*, 1275—1282.

Hiki, S. (1967): Correlation between increments of voice pitch and glottal sound intensity. J. Acoust. Soc. Jpn. *23*, 20—22.

Hiki, S., Imaizumi, S., Hirano, M., Matsushita, H., Kakita, Y. (1976): Acoustical analysis for voice disorders. Conference Record, 1976 IEEE International Conference on Acoustics, Speech, and Signal Processing. Rome, N.Y.: Canterbury Press.

Hirano, M. (1975): Phonosurgery. Basic and clinical investigations. Otologia (Fukuoka) *21*, 239—440.

Hirano, M., Kakita, Y., Matsushita, H., Hiki, S., Imaizumi, S. (1977a): Correlation between parameters related to vocal vibration and acoustical parameters in voice disorders. Pract. Otol. (Kyoto) *70*, 393—403.

Hirano, M., Kakita, Y., Matsushita, H., Hiki, S., Imaizumi, S. (1977b): Psychoacoustic parameters in voice disorders. Pract. Otol. (Kyoto) *70*, 525—531.

Hirano, M., Matsushita, H., Hiki, S., Kakita, Y. (1976): Acoustic analysis for voice disorders. A basic conception for the use of acoustic measurements for the diagnosis in voice disorders. Pract. Otol. (Kyoto) *69*, 267—271.

Imaizumi, S., Hiki, S., Hirano, M., Matsushita, H. (1980): Analysis of pathological voices with a sound spectrograph. J. Acoust. Soc. Jpn. *36*, 9—16.

Isshiki, N., Yanagihara, N., Morimoto, M. (1966): Approach to the objective diagnosis of hoarseness. Folia Phoniat. *18*, 393—400.

Iwata, S. (1972): Periodicities of pitch perturbations in normal and pathological larynges. Laryngoscope *82*, 87—96.

Iwata, S., von Leden, H. (1969): Acoustic studies and computer techniques in the diagnosis of laryngeal disorders. Oto-Rhino-Laryngology (Proceeding of the Ninth International Congress), pp. 286—290.

Iwata, S., von Leden, H. (1970): Pitch perturbations in normal and pathologic voices. Folia Phoniat. *22*, 413—424.

Kakita, Y., Hirano, M., Matsushita, H., Hiki, S., Imaizumi, S. (1977a): Acoustical parameters relevant to diagnosis in voice disorders. Pract. Otol. (Kyoto) *70*, 269—276.

Kakita, Y., Hirano, M., Matsushita, H., Hiki, S., Imaizumi, S. (1977b): Differentiation of laryngeal diseases using acoustical analysis. Pract. Otol. (Kyoto) *70*, 729—739.

Kirikae, I., Matsuzaki, T., Funasaka, S. (1965): An experimental study on pertubations in vocal pitch. J. Otolaryngol. Jpn. *68*, 364—374.

Kitajima, K., Tanabe, M., Isshiki, N. (1975): Pitch perturbation in normal and pathologic voice. Studia Phonologica *9*, 25—32.

Koike, Y. (1969): Vowel amplitude modulations in patients with laryngeal diseases. J. Acoust. Soc. Amer. *45*, 839—844.

Koike, Y. (1973): Application of some acoustic measures for the evaluation of laryngeal dysfunction. Studia Phonologica *7*, 17—23.

Koike, Y., Markel, J. D. (1975): Application of inverse filtering for detecting laryngeal pathology. Ann. Otol. *84*, 117—124.

Koike, Y., Takahashi, H. (1971): Glottal parameters and some acoustic measures in patients with laryngeal pathology. Studia Phonologica 7, 45–50.

Kreul, J., Hecker, M. H. L. (1971): Description of the speech of patients with cancer of the vocal folds. Part II. Judgements of age and voice quality. J. Acoust. Soc. Amer. 49, 1283–1287.

Laguaite, J., Wakdrop, W. F. (1963): Acoustic analysis of fundamental frequency of voice before and after therapy. N. Z. Speech Therapist J. 18, 23–25.

Lieberman, P. (1961): Perturbation in vocal pitch. J. Acoust. Soc. Amer. 33, 597–603.

Lieberman, P. (1962): Pitch perturbation of normal and pathologic laryngeal. Fourth International Congress on Acoustics, pp. 1–4.

Lieberman, P. (1963): Some acoustic measures of the fundamental periodicity of normal and pathologic larynges. J. Acoust. Soc. Amer. 35, 344–353.

Makhoul, J. (1975): Linear prediction: A tutorial review. Proceedings of the IEEE 63, 561–580.

Markel, J. D., Gray, A. H., jr. (1976): Linear Prediction of Speech. New York: Springer.

Miller, N. J. (1974): Pitch detection by data reduction. IEEE Symposium on Speech Recognition, pp. 122–130.

Monsen, R. B. (1979): The use of a reflectionless tube to assess vocal function. NIH Conference on Assessment of Vocal Pathology.

Nessel, E. (1960): Über das Tonfrequenzspektrum der pathologisch veränderten Stimme. Acta Otolaryngol. 157, 1–45.

Ono, H., Saito, S., Okazaki, T., Ookawa, H., Ozawa, S. (1975): Observation of the vocal cord vibration using online computer system and clinical application. J. Acoust. Soc. Jpn. 31, 228–231.

Ono, H., Tamura, H., Saito, S., Kitahara, S., Suzuki, Y. (1973): Observation of the vocal cord vibration by glottal waves and its clinical applications. J. Otolaryngol. Jpn. 76, 495–500.

Sondhi, M. M. (1975): Measurement of the glottal waveform. J. Acoust. Soc. Amer. 57, 228–232.

Takahashi, H., Koike, Y. (1975): Some perceptual dimensions and acoustical correlates of pathologic voices. Acta Otolaryngol. 338, 1–24.

Takasugi, T., Nakatsui, M., Suzuki, J. (1970): Observation of glottal waveform from speech waves. J. Acoust. Soc. Jpn. 26, 141–149.

Wendahl, R. W. (1963): Laryngeal analog synthesis of harch voice quality. Folia Phoniat. 15, 241–250.

Wendahl, R. W. (1966): Laryngeal analog synthesis of jitter and shimmer auditory parameters of harshness. Folia Phoniat. 18, 98–108.

von Leden, H., Koike, Y. (1970): Detection of laryngeal disease by computer technique. Arch. Otolaryngol. 91, 3–10.

Yanagihara, N. (1967a): Significance of harmonic changes and noise components in hoarseness. J. Sp. Hear. Res. 10, 531–541.

Yanagihara, N. (1967b): Hoarseness: Investigation of the physiological mechanisms. Ann. Otol. 76, 472–489.

# Psycho-Acoustic Evaluation of Voice  6

The human ear has a surprising capability to identify and discriminate varying sound complexes. One can often identify the speaker simply by listening to the voice. Well-trained voice clinicians are frequently able to determine the causative pathologies on the basis of the psycho-acoustic impression of abnormal voices (Takahashi, 1974; Takahashi *et al.*, 1974; Hirano, 1975). This appears to be analogous to the auscultation of heart sounds and respiratory sounds by physicians.

The nature of the pathological voice has been classified and described in terms of its auditory impression: hoarseness, harshness, breathiness, dry hoarseness, wet hoarseness, rough hoarseness, and so on. The definition of these terms, however, has often been controversial and not always common to all voice specialists. Standardization of psycho-acoustic evaluation of the pathological voice and of the terminology is required. Such standardization and its subsequent clinical application appear to call for detailed investigations with the use of sophisticated psychometric techniques and a reasonable international agreement.

In this chapter, some attempts relevant to this goal are reviewed.

## A. Studies with Semantic Differential Techniques

The semantic differential techniques proposed by Osgood *et al.* (1957) have been utilized for psychometric studies of pathological voices by two groups of investigators.

### 1. Isshiki Classification of the Hoarse Voice

Isshiki (1966) applied the semantic differential technique to factor analysis of hoarseness. He selected 17 pairs of polar-opposite adjectives as the scales: three pairs representing an evaluation factor, three pairs representing a potency factor, three pairs representing an activity factor, and eight pairs being apparently relevant to describe hoarseness. Sixteen recorded samples of a hoarse voice (five Japanese vowels) varying in quality, degree and genesis were analysed.

On the basis of the analysis of the data, Isshiki reported that hoarse voice consisted of at least four factors. The first factor, exceedingly dominant over the other factors, appeared to correspond closely with the voice quality which was expressed as "rough, rumbling, or rattling". This factor was arbitrarily referred to as factor "R". The second factor was related to the voice quality which was described as "breathy". It was arbitrarily called factor "B". The third factor appeared to be closest to what had been expressed as "asthenic". It was referred to as factor "A". The fourth factor indicated slight degrees of hoarseness. It was referred to as "semi-normality", "close to normal" and abbreviated "N". Since this factor was linked with the degree of hoarseness, it was expressed as factor "D" in a later publication (Isshiki et al., 1969).

The use of all the 17 scales in analyzing hoarse voices is too laborious and time-consuming to be utilized in outpatient clinics. Therefore, Isshiki and his co-workers proposed a simplified version (Isshiki et al., 1969; Isshiki and Takeuchi, 1970). It consisted of an evaluation of hoarseness with respect to the four factors "R, B, A and D", using a four point grading (0 = normal, 1 = slight, 2 = fair, 3 = extreme). They reported a very close correlation between the original method and the simplified version.

Hiroto (1967) made a sound spectrographic analytical study of the 16 voice samples which had been used for the semantic differential study by Isshiki. The hoarse voice of a breathy nature was characterized by noise ranging from low to high frequencies and poor harmonic components. The rough type of the hoarse voice presented with fluctuations in the amplitude and the fundamental frequency. The asthenic variety of the hoarse voice was chiefly characterized by a weak intensity. Hiroto also pointed out that low-pitched voices tended to sound rough, whereas high-pitched voices sounded breathy or asthenic.

Isshiki et al. (1969) described that the voice best represented by factor R is characterized by a great pitch perturbation, while the voice represented by factor B is distinguished by a marked noise component and a greatly reduced or negligible harmonic component.

## 2. Takahashi — Koike's Investigation

Takahashi and Koike (1976) carried out a detailed investigation of some of the perceptual dimensions of pathological voices and related these to selected acoustical correlates.

They adopted two sets of test stimuli. The first set of stimuli consisted of samples of the vowel [a] tape-recorded from 24 subjects: nine normal persons and 15 patients with various laryngeal diseases. The second set of stimuli consisted of nine synthesized vowel samples, having three different fundamental frequencies at three intensity levels. They employed the semantic differential technique for the perceptual study. Twelve pairs of polar-opposite adjectives were selected as the scales for the listener's judgements: the first four pairs represented an evaluation factor, the second four a potency factor, and the other four an activity factor. In addition to the psycho-acoustic assessment described above, two listeners who were laryngologists evaluated all the voice samples with regard to their quality of breathiness and roughness. In addition, Takahashi and Koike utilized measurements of the fundamental frequency, the frequency perturbation quotient (FPQ) and the amplitude perturbation quotient (APQ), as their acoustic correlates.

They analyzed the data with two methods, that is, D-method of factoring and Lawley's maximum likelihood method with Kaiser's varimax rotation.

In the D-method, dimension I was related to both the breathy and rough scores as well as to the FPQ and APQ. This dimension was of an evaluative nature. Dimension II was reasonably related to the sensation of loudness. Dimension III was correlated positively with the fundamental frequency and was also related to pitch sensation. Dimension IV was correlated with the breathy score and APQ, and seemed to be associated with the perception of breathiness.

In the maximum likelihood method, factor I was inversely related to FPQ and APQ, suggesting that it was of an evaluative nature. Factor II was correlated with the fundamental frequency and, therefore, was related to pitch sensation. Factor III was apparently related to the degree of loudness. The nature of factor IV was not very clear.

On the basis of these results, Takahashi and Koike felt that the four dominant factors extracted in Isshiki's study, using the same procedure as theirs, should correspond to the dimensions discussed in their report. They further stated that Isshiki's terms, such as "rough" (R), "breathy" (B), "asthenic" (A), and "degree" (D), had no tenable basis and was misleading.

Yoshida (1979) conducted psychometric and acoustical analysis of 30 pathological voice samples obtained from 10 patients with vocal fold polyps, 10 patients with vocal fold paralysis, and 10 patients with carcinoma of the vocal fold. He also used the semantic differential technique. His results agreed with those of Takahashi and Koike.

# B. "GRBAS" Scale for Evaluating the Hoarse Voice

The Committee for Phonatory Function Tests of the Japan Society of Logopedics and Phoniatrics proposed the "GRBAS" scale for evaluating hoarseness. It consists of five scales: grade (G), rough (R), breathy (B), asthenic (A), and strained (S).

The first scale G represents the degree of hoarseness or voice abnormality. It corresponds to the factor of evaluative nature obtained by the semantic differential technique. The remaining four scales represent different aspects of voice abnormality. Scale R represents a psycho-acoustic impression of the irregularity of vocal fold vibrations. It corresponds to the irregular fluctuations in the fundamental frequency and/or the amplitude of the glottal source sound. Scale B represents a psycho-acoustic impression of the extent of air leakage through the glottis. It is related to turbulence. Scale A denotes weakness or lack of power in the voice. It is related to a weak intensity of the glottal source sound and/or a lack of higher harmonics. Scale S represents a psycho-acoustic impression of a hyperfunctional state of phonation. It is related to an abnormally high fundamental frequency, noise in the high frequency range, and/or richness in high frequency harmonics.

Hoarse voices can be evaluated with the use of these five scales. A four-point grading is used for each scale: "0" non-hoarse or normal, "1" slight, "2" moderate, and "3" extreme. The results of the evaluation are, therefore, described as $G_1 R_1 B_1 A_0 S_0$, $G_3 R_3 B_3 A_0 S_3$, $G_2 R_1 B_3 A_2 S_0$, and so on.

Since the evaluation with the use of GRBAS scale is subjective, the examiner must possess a trained ear. For this purpose, the Committee for Phonatory Function Tests of the Japan Society of Logopedics and Phoniatrics has made a standard tape which has typical voice samples represented by GRBAS scale. The Committee feels that the psycho-acoustic evaluation using the GRBAS scale is not an absolute method but needs to be improved upon.

# References

Hirano, M. (1975): Phonosurgery. Basic and clinical investigations. Otologia (Fukuoka) 27, 239–440.

Hiroto, I. (1967): Hoarseness. Viewpoints of voice physiology. Jpn. J. Logop. Phoniat. 8, 9–15.

Isshiki, N. (1966): Classification of hoarseness. Jpn. J. Logop. Phoniat. 7, 15–21.

Isshiki, N., Okamura, H., Tanabe, M., Morimoto, M. (1969): Differential diagnosis of hoarseness. Folia Phoniat. 21, 9–19.

Isshiki, N., Takeuchi, Y. (1970): Factor analysis of hoarseness. Studia Phonologica 5, 37–44.

Osgood, C. E., Suci, G. J., Tannenbaum, P. H. H. (1957): The Measurement of Meaning. Urbana, Ill.: University of Illinois Press.

Takahashi, H. (1974): Significance of perceptual study of pathological voices. Pract. Otol. (Kyoto) 67, 949–953.

Takahashi, H., Koike, Y. (1976): Some perceptual dimensions and acoustical correlates of pathologic voices. Acta Otolaryngol., Suppl. 338, 1–24.

Takahashi, H., Yoshida, M., Oshima, T., Sakamoto, K., Tsumura, S., Yamazaki, T. (1974): On the differential diagnosis of laryngeal pathologies through the perceptual impression of the voices. Pract. Otol. (Kyoto) 67, 1377–1385.

Yoshida, M. (1979): Study on perceptive and acoustical classification of pathologic voices. Pract. Otol. (Kyoto) 72, 249–287.

# Examination of Phonatory Ability 7

The term phonatory ability implies such abilities in voice production as how long one can sustain phonation, what range of fundamental frequencies one can cover, how one can control the vocal register, what range of vocal intensity one can produce, how efficiently one can convert the aerodynamic energy to acoustic energy (glottal efficiency), and so on. In this chapter, some important tests to evaluate phonatory ability are described.

## A. Maximum Phonation Time

### 1. Method of Measurement

The subject is instructed to sustain vowel /a/ as long as possible following deep inspiration. The phonation is made at the fundamental frequency and intensity level comfortable for the subject. In some particular cases, such as in examining a singer, the fundamental frequency and/or intensity level may be controlled. The duration of the maximum sustained phonation is called the maximum phonation time (MPT). Measurements are made three times and the greatest value is adopted (Sawashima, 1966). Measurements are usually done with the subject standing. There is, however, no significant difference in MPT in the standing and sitting positions (Sawashima, 1966).

### 2. Normal Values for Maximum Phonation Time

Table 7.1 presents normal values for MPT reported by several investigators. The average is greater for males (25—35 sec) than females (15—25 sec). The upper limit of the critical region is greater for males than females, whereas the lower limit does not

Table 7.1. *Normal values of maximum phonation time (in sec) in adults*

| Author(s) | N | | Average* | | Confidence limit | Critical region | Range |
|---|---|---|---|---|---|---|---|
| Hayashi (1940) | M | 20 | | 22 | | | |
| | | | /i/ | 25 | | | |
| Suzuki (1944) | M | 21 | | 24.8 | | | 15 —37 |
| | F | 19 | | 17.4 | | | 10 —24 |
| Nishikawa (1962) | Singer | 10 | | | | | 19 —38 |
| | M | 10 | | | | | 16 —29 |
| | F | 10 | | | | | 12 —21 |
| Ptacek and Sander | M | 40 | I | 24.7 | | | 13.6—41.7 |
| (1963) | | | II | 25.7 | | | 14.3—48.0 |
| | | | III | 24.9 | | | 12.3—59.0 |
| | F | 40 | I | 16.8 | | | 9.3—34.0 |
| | | | II | 16.7 | | | 9.2—29.8 |
| | | | III | 17.9 | | | 8.4—39.7 |
| Sawashima (1966) | M | 70 | | 29.7 | | 13.9—51.4 | |
| | F | 78 | | 20.3 | | 9.0—36.2 | |
| Yanagihara *et al.* (1966) | M | 11 | | 30.2 | | | 20.4—50.7 |
| | F | 11 | | 22.5 | | | 16.4—32.7 |
| Isshiki *et al.* (1967) | M | 5 | | 31 | | | 22 —51 |
| | F | 5 | | 17 | | | 9 —36 |
| Hirano *et al.* (1968) | M | 25 | | 34.6 | | 30.2—39.4 | 15.0—62.3 | |
| | F | 25 | | 25.7 | | 22.9—28.7 | 14.3—40.4 | |
| Shigemori (1977) | M | 25 | | 30.1 | | 25.9—34.5 | 12.0—56.2 | 15.8—66.6 |
| | F | 25 | | 17.0 | | 15.2—18.9 | 9.0—27.5 | 9.4—26.2 |

* Unless otherwise noted measurements were made on the vowel /a/. Roman numerals refer to the trial number.

Table 7.2. *Normal values of maximum phonation time (in sec) in children (Shigemori, 1977)*

| Grade level | | Average | Confidence limit (95%) | Critical region (95%) | Range |
|---|---|---|---|---|---|
| | male | 14.2 | 12.7—15.7 | 7.6—22.7 | 9.6—22.0 |
| 1st grade | female | 13.1 | 11.8—14.4 | 7.2—20.6 | 9.0—20.6 |
| | total | 13.6 | 12.6—14.6 | 7.6—21.4 | 9.0—22.0 |
| | male | 16.2 | 14.9—17.5 | 10.2—23.6 | 10.0—21.2 |
| 3rd grade | female | 15.2 | 13.9—16.6 | 9.1—23.0 | 9.2—20.6 |
| | total | 15.7 | 14.8—16.7 | 9.8—23.1 | 9.2—21.2 |
| | male | 19.2 | 17.4—21.1 | 10.8—29.9 | 13.0—32.8 |
| 5th grade | female | 16.3 | 14.4—18.3 | 7.9—27.7 | 9.4—26.0 |
| | total | 17.7 | 16.4—19.1 | 9.2—28.9 | 9.4—32.8 |
| | male | 23.7 | 20.3—27.4 | 9.0—45.5 | 10.8—46.5 |
| 7th grade | female | 19.8 | 17.7—22.2 | 10.0—33.0 | 13.6—34.8 |
| | total | 21.7 | 19.7—23.9 | 9.4—39.2 | 10.8—46.5 |

differ markedly between males and females. Clinically, MPT values smaller than 10 sec should be considered to be abnormal.

Shigemori (1977) investigated MPT in school children (Table 7.2). The MPT was found to increase with age. The differences between males and females were not significant except in the seventh grade children.

## 3. Maximum Phonation Time in Pathological States

MPT is decreased in many pathological states of the larynx, especially in cases with incompetent glottal closure. Tables 7.3 and 7.4 present MPT in pathological cases reported by Hirano *et al.* (1968) and Shigemori (1977) respectively. An abnormally short MPT was frequently found in cases of recurrent laryngeal nerve paralysis. Out of the 113 cases of unilateral paralysis of the recurrent laryngeal nerve studied by Shigemori, the paretic vocal fold was fixed in the intermediate or in the paramedian position in 63 cases whilst it was fixed in the median position or had an

Table 7.3. *Maximum phonation time (in sec) in pathological states (Hirano et al., 1968)*

|  |  | Critical region | |  |
|---|---|---|---|---|
|  |  | Confidence limit | |  |
| Neoplasm (10) | 4 | 5 | 1 |  |
| Polyp (10) | 6 | 3 | 1 |  |
| Nodule (8) |  | 6 | 2 |  |
| Granuloma (5) |  | 3 | 1 | 1 |
| Laryngitis (5) | 2 | 3 |  |  |
| Paralysis (13) | 10 | 2 | 1 |  |
| Trauma (1) | 1 |  |  |  |
| Web (1) | 1 |  |  |  |
| Throiditis (2) |  | 2 |  |  |
| Mutation (1) |  | 1 |  |  |
| Virilization (1) |  | 1 |  |  |
| Spastic dysphonia (8) | 3 | 4 | 1 |  |
| Hysteric dysphonia (3) | 2 | 1 |  |  |
| Phonasthenia (1) | 1 |  |  |  |

Table 7.4. *Maximum phonation time (in sec) in pathological states (Shigemori, 1977)*

|  |  | N | MPT $\leq$ 10.0 sec | Range |
|---|---|---|---|---|
| Recurrent laryngeal | Unilateral | 113 | 73 (65%) | 1.9—42.0 |
| nerve paralysis | Bilateral | 9 | 5 (56%) | 2.4—20.0 |
| Sulcus vocalis |  | 26 | 8 (29%) | 3.8—42.0 |
| Laryngitis |  | 59 | 10 (17%) | 4.0—38.0 |
| Nodule, Polyp |  | 182 | 44 (24%) | 1.7—48.8 |
| Polypoid vocal fold |  | 36 | 11 (31%) | 4.0—38.8 |
| Benign tumor |  | 28 | 5 (23%) | 7.0—39.6 |
| Epithelial hyperplasia |  | 14 | 0 | 10.2—49.2 |
| Carcinoma |  | 34 | 6 (18%) | 5.4—41.8 |

impaired mobility in 50 cases. In the former group, 48 cases (76 per cent) presented with MPT's shorter than 10 sec. In the latter group, MPT was shorter than 10 sec in 25 cases (50 per cent).

Shigemori (1977) reported that the MPT is valuable for monitoring the effects of surgical treatment in selected disorders of the larynx, especially in recurrent laryngeal nerve paralysis, and, to a certain extent, in cases of sulcus vocalis, nodules, polyps and polypoid vocal folds.

# B. Frequency Range of Phonation

## 1. Terminology

The range of the fundamental frequency of voice that one can produce is called the frequency range of phonation (FRP). It is also referred to as vocal range, vocal pitch range, phonational range or phonational frequency range. Its extent is from the lowest tone in the modal register to the highest in falsetto. The tones in the vocal fry register are not included. The range is usually described in semitones.

There are two kinds of FRP, the physiological frequency range of phonation (PFRP) and the musical, or singing, frequency range of phonation (MFRP). The former applies to voice of any quality whereas the latter applies to the voice with musically acceptable qualities. As a clinical test, PFRP is usually measured. MFRP is important to evaluate singing ability.

## 2. Method of Measurement

The most popular method employs a piano or an organ. The subject is instructed to sing ascending musical scales, starting with a tone which can be sung easily in the modal register, accompanied by the instrument. The highest physiological tone (HPT) is determined by matching the vocal tone with the tone produced by the

Table 7.5. *Pitch names and fundamental frequency*

| | $C_0$ $(C_2)$ | $C_1$ $(C_1)$ | $C_2$ $(C\ )$ | $C_3$ $(c^0)$ | $C_4$ $(c^1)$ | $C_5$ $(c^2)$ | $C_6$ $(c^3)$ | $C_7$ $(c^4)$ | Quotient |
|---|---|---|---|---|---|---|---|---|---|
| c | 16,35 | 32,70 | 65,41 | 130,81 | 261,63 | 523,25 | 1046,50 | 2093,00 | $= 1,000000$ |
| $c^\sharp$, $d^b$ | 71,32 | 34,64 | 69,29 | 138,59 | 277,18 | 554,37 | 1108,73 | 2217,46 | $\sqrt[12]{2} = 1,05946$ |
| d | 18,35 | 36,71 | 73,42 | 146,84 | 293,67 | 587,33 | 1174,66 | 2349,31 | $\sqrt[12]{2^2} = 1,12246$ |
| $d^\sharp$, $e^b$ | 19,45 | 38,89 | 77,78 | 155,56 | 311,13 | 622,25 | 1244,51 | 2489,01 | $\sqrt[12]{2^3} = 1,18921$ |
| e | 20,60 | 41,41 | 82,40 | 164,81 | 329,63 | 659,25 | 1318,51 | 2637,02 | $\sqrt[12]{2^4} = 1,25992$ |
| f | 21,83 | 43,65 | 87,31 | 174,61 | 349,23 | 698,46 | 1396,91 | 2793,82 | $\sqrt[12]{2^5} = 1,33484$ |
| $f^\sharp$, $g^b$ | 23,13 | 46,25 | 92,50 | 185,00 | 369,99 | 739,98 | 1479,98 | 2959,95 | $\sqrt[12]{2^6} = 1,41421$ |
| g | 24,50 | 49,00 | 98,00 | 196,00 | 392,00 | 783,99 | 1567,98 | 3135,95 | $\sqrt[12]{2^7} = 1,49831$ |
| $g^\sharp$, $a^b$ | 25,96 | 51,92 | 103,83 | 207,65 | 415,30 | 830,61 | 1661,22 | 3322,43 | $\sqrt[12]{2^8} = 1,58740$ |
| a | 27,50 | 55,00 | 110,00 | 220,00 | 440,00 | 880,00 | 1760,00 | 3520,00 | $\sqrt[12]{2^9} = 1,68179$ |
| $a^\sharp$, $b^b$ | 29,14 | 58,27 | 116,54 | 233,08 | 466,16 | 923,33 | 1864,65 | 3729,30 | $\sqrt[12]{2^{10}} = 1,78180$ |
| b | 30,86 | 61,73 | 123,47 | 246,94 | 493,88 | 987,77 | 1975,53 | 3951,06 | $\sqrt[12]{2^{11}} = 1,88775$ |

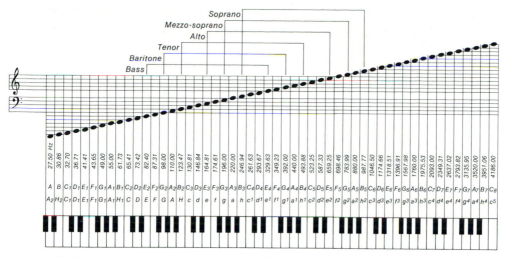

Fig. 7.1. Presentation of pitch names on a staff notation and a key board of a piano

instrument. In the same manner, the lowest physiological tone (LPT) is determined while singing descending scales. The highest and the lowest musical tones (HMT and LMT) are also determined, if necessary, during these procedures. The PFRP corresponds to the difference between HPT and LPT, and is expressed in semitones. HPT and LPT, as well as PFRP, are described. When the singing ability is assessed, HMT, LMT and MFRP are also recorded.

Many kinds of "pitch meters" are now available for measurement of HPT, LPT and PFRP. When a pitch meter is used, the HPT and LPT are expressed in Hz. In such cases however, it is not advisable to present PFRP in Hz by subtracting LPT (in Hz) from HPT (in Hz). For example, the interval of 220 Hz between $A_3$ (220 Hz) and $A_4$ (440 Hz) corresponds to 12 semitones whereas the interval of 220 Hz between $A_4$ (440 Hz) and $E_5$ (659 Hz) corresponds to seven semitones. The fundamental frequency of each pitch name is presented in Table 7.5; Table 7.5 is useful for converting the frequency interval of any two fundamental frequencies into a semitone interval.

Fig. 7.1 shows pitch names on a staff notation and a key board of a piano.

## 3. Normal Values of Frequency Range of Phonation

Table 7.6 presents LPT, HPT and PFRP of normal adults reported by several investigators. The average PFRP is approximately three octaves (36 semitones) for males. For females, it is approximately three octaves in American literature and approximately two and a half octaves in Japanese literature. It should be noted, however, that there are large individual variations in PFRP.

With regard to the FRP in children, there are two conflicting opinions reviewed by van Oordt and Drost (1963). Gutsmann holds the view that FRP develops gradually from birth. The first cries of the newborn lie around $A_4$ (440 Hz), after

Table 7.6. *Average lowest physiological tone (LPT), highest physiological tone (HPT) and physiological frequency range of phonation (PFRP) in normal adults*

| Author(s) | Sex | LPT | HPT | PFRP in semitones |
|---|---|---|---|---|
| Ihda (1940) | Male | D$_2^{\sharp}$ | D$_5$ | 35 (30−39)* |
|  | Female | D$_3^{\sharp}$ | G$_5$ | 28 (24−31) |
| Sawashima (1968) | Male | C$_2^{\sharp}$ | D$_5$ | 37 (32−43)* |
|  | Female | C$_3$ | G$_5$ | 30 (26−34) |
| Hollien *et al.* (1971) | Male | E$_2$ | F$_5$ | 38 (13−55)** |
|  | Female | D$_3$ | D$_6$ | 37 (23−50) |
| Coleman *et al.* (1977) | Male |  |  | 37 (29−44)** |
|  | Female |  |  | 37 (31−42) |

\* S.D. in parenthesis, ** range in parenthesis.

which FRP increases steadily with age. Just before the adolescent voice changes, FRP has reached one and a half octaves. Hartlieb reported that FRP of at least two octaves is reached during the first year of life and FRP, LPT and HPT remain the same until the voice changes at adolescence. According to van Oordt and Drost, Hartlieb's theory is partially correct as far as PFRP is concerned, but Gutzmann's concept holds true for MFRP.

The average MFRP for different voice types is shown in Fig. 7.1.

Böhme and Hecker (1970) conducted an extensive investigation of MFRP with 632 subjects with their age ranging from six to 90 years. Their results are shown in Figs. 7.2, 7.3, and 7.4. According to these workers, the entire course of the age-dependent changes in MFRP can be divided into three phases: (1) expansion of MFRP up to the end of adolescent voice change, (2) constant MFRP in adults from late teens to about 60 years, and (3) progressive decrease in MFRP after the 60th year of life. During the second phase, MFRP is measured to be approximately two octaves.

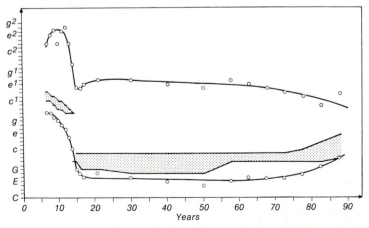

Fig. 7.2. Highest and lowest musical tones (HMT, LMT) and mean speaking frequency (MSF) shown as a function of age in males (Böhme and Hecker, 1970)

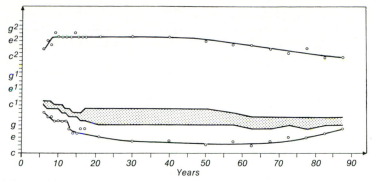

Fig. 7.3. Highest and lowest musical tones (HMT, LMT) and mean speaking frequency (MSF) shown as a function of age in females (Böhme and Hecker, 1970)

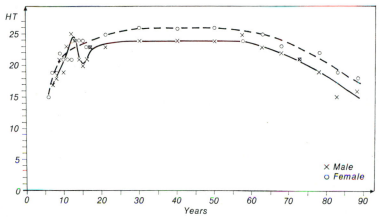

Fig. 7.4. Average musical frequency range of phonation (MFRP) in semitones shown as a function of age (Böhme and Hecker, 1970)

## 4. Frequency Range of Phonation in Pathological States

Sawashima (1968) investigated LPT, HPT and PFRP in various cases of vocal fold abnormalities. Fig. 7.5 presents his results. In all the disorders shown here, HPT tends to be lowered. In laryngeal paralysis and sulcus vocalis, LPT becomes high resulting in a small PFRP. LPT is lowered in the cases of polypoid vocal fold and of virilism caused by an anabolic hormone.

## C. Speaking Fundamental Frequency

During speech, the fundamental frequency of phonation varies. This range of variation is called the speech range or speech frequency range (SFR). The average fundamental frequency during speech or the most frequent fundamental frequency during speech is referred to as the mean speaking fundamental frequency, or

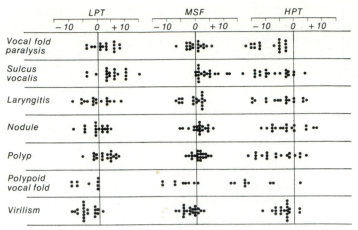

Fig. 7.5. Highest and lowest physiological tones *(HPT, LPT)* and mean speaking frequency *(MSF)* in pathological states (Sawashima, 1968)

simply, the mean speaking frequency (MSF). At present, MSF is measured as a clinical test value. The clinical significance of SFR awaits further investigation.

MSF may not always represent phonatory ability. It is, however, related to FRP, and is therefore described in this chapter.

## 1. Method of Measurement

Several types of speech samples have been used for the measurement of MSF:

(1) Habitual speech in conversation
(2) Reading a given passage
(3) Counting
(4) Sustained vowel at the end of a given word
(5) Sustained single vowel with minimum effort

Differences in MSF between these different kinds of speech samples are debatable. For example, Schultz—Coulon (1975) reported that MSF during habitual speech was significantly lower than during reading and counting. On the other hand, Nishiyama (1969) found no significant difference in MSF during habitual speech, reading or sustained single vowel.

MSF is estimated subjectively by matching or it is determined objectively with the use of an instrument such as pitch meter. For more precise measurement, fundamental frequency histograms are obtained with the aid of a computer.

## 2. Normal Values of Mean Speaking Frequency

Table 7.7 presents MSF of adults reported by several investigators. The average MSF appears to lie between $A_2$ and $C_3$ (range, $F_2^\# - D_3$) for males and between $G_3$ and $A_3^\#$ (range $F_3^\# - C_4$) for females.

Table 7.7. *Mean speaking frequency (MSF) in normal adults*

| Author(s) | | Sex | Average | Range |
|---|---|---|---|---|
| Ihda (1940) | | male<br>female | $A_2$<br>$G_3^\sharp$ | $G_2$–$B_2$<br>$F_3^\sharp$–$A_3$ |
| Sawashima (1968) | | male<br>female | $C_3$<br>$A_3^\sharp$ | $A_2^\sharp$–$D_3$<br>$A_3$–$C_4$ |
| Böhme and Hecker (1970) | | male<br>female | | $F_2^\sharp$–$B_2$<br>$G_3$–$B_3$ |
| Schultz – Coulon (1975) | Reading | male<br>female | 117 Hz, $A_2^\sharp$<br>208 Hz, $G_3^\sharp$ | |
| | Counting | male<br>female | 110 Hz, $A_2$<br>198 Hz, $G_3$ | |
| | Speech | male<br>female | 107 Hz, $<A_2$<br>191 Hz, $F_3^\sharp$–$G_3$ | |

The age dependent variations of MSF reported by Böhme and Hecker (1970) are shown in Figs. 7.2 and 7.3 MSF decreases with age up to the end of adolescence. A marked lowering of MSF takes place during adolescence in men. In advanced age, MSF becomes higher in men but is slightly lowered in women. Hollien and Shipp (1972) investigated MSF of 175 males and reported a progressive lowering of MSF from 20 to 40 years of age with a rise in the level from 60 to 80.

MSF usually lies in the lowest fourth of PFRP and in the bottom third of MFRP.

## 3. Mean Speaking Frequency in Pathological States

Sawashima (1968) reported a rise in MSF in cases of sulcus vocalis and a fall in MSF in cases of polypoid vocal fold and virilism (Fig. 7.5). Very high MSF values can result from disturbances of mutation in males.

Besides exceptionally high or low MSF values, monotonic speaking frequency (monotone or monopitch), "breaks" of fundamental frequency (pitch breaks) and stereotyped inflections of the speaking frequency are important manifestations of voice disorders.

# D. Vocal Register

There are three major categories of vocal register: vocal fry, modal register and falsetto. The classification is based upon the quality of the glottal sound determined by the vibratory pattern of the vocal folds. The modal register can be further divided into three: the chest, mid and head registers. In general, the vocal register is closely related to the fundamental frequency of phonation: Along the fundamental frequency from low to high, the register is put in the order of vocal fry, chest, mid, head, and falsetto. There are, however, frequency ranges where two or more registers overlap.

From a clinical point of view, the capability to produce voices in different registers, especially, in both the modal register and falsetto, is important. In evaluating singing ability, one should find out if the register shifts are made without abrupt audible changes in voice quality. The frequency range of each register should also be examined.

## E. Intensity Range of Phonation

The range of the intensity of voice one can produce is defined as the intensity range of phonation (IRP). Empirically, it is well known that disorders of vocal intensity constitute one of the important components of voice disorder. However, measurement of vocal intensity has not proved as popular as that of fundamental frequency in voice clinics. This may be attributed to the need for sophisticated instruments for intensity measurements and also to the lack of standardized methods. Fortunately, recent advances in technology have made it possible to measure the vocal intensity using rather simple and inexpensive instruments.

The Committee for Phonatory Function Tests of the Japan Society of Logopedics and Phoniatrics proposed that vocal intensity should be measured at a distance of 20 cm, that the intensity should be expressed in sound pressure level (re: 0.0002 dyne/cm²), and that a soundproof room is desirable for the measurement.

IRP varies with the fundamental frequency (Damsté, 1970; Komiyama, 1972; Coleman *et al.*, 1977). It is greatest at the middle frequency range and becomes smaller as the lowest and highest tones are approached. According to Coleman *et al.* (1977), the average IRP (in SPL re: 0.0002 dyne/cm$^2$) at a single fundamental frequency is 54.8 dB for male and 51 dB for female subjects.

## F. Fundamental Frequency-Intensity Profile

A graphic presentation of the fundamental frequency-intensity profile was proposed by Damsté (1970), Komiyama (1972) and Coleman *et al.* (1977). Fig. 7.6A, B, C, and D demonstrate examples of the profile reported by these authors. The graph was named "phonetogram" by Damsté and "phonogram" by Komiyama. They suggested that the graph could be used in evaluating vocal function in various disorders as well as in monitoring the effects of treatment.

## G. Glottal Efficiency

The glottal efficiency (GE) is defined as the ratio of the acoustic power at the level of the glottis ($I_{GL}$) to the subglottal power ($W_{SUB}$) as shown in the following equation:

$$GE = \frac{I_{GL}}{W_{SUB}} \tag{1}$$

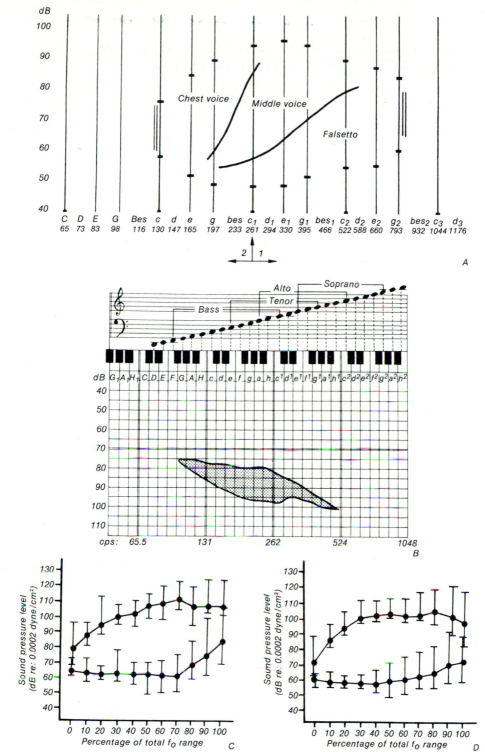

Fig. 7.6. Fundamental frequency-intensity profile. *A* "phonetogram" by Damsté (1970). *B* "phonogram" by Komiyama (1972). *C* fundamental frequency-SPL level profile for males by Coleman *et al.* (1977). *D* fundamental frequency-SPL level profile for females by Coleman *et al.* (1977)

Since the subglottal power is a product of the subglottal pressure ($P_{SUB}$) and the airflow rate (MFR), the glottal efficiency is also expressed as:

$$GE = \frac{I_{GL}}{P_{SUB} \times MFR} \tag{2}$$

Since it is difficult to measure $I_{GL}$ clinically, GE has not been used as clinical test. Several alternatives have been proposed.

## 1. Ratio of Radiated Acoustic Power to Subglottal Power

The radiated acoustic power, *i.e.* the intensity of phonation measured at a certain distance from the mouth (I), can be used as a substitute for $I_{GL}$ in equation (2). The ratio shown in equation (3) may be regarded as an efficiency of the glottis-vocal tract system (GVTE).

$$GVTE = \frac{I}{P_{SUB} \times MFR} \tag{3}$$

If the vocal tract shape is kept constant, as in phonation through a tube held in the mouth, GVTE reflects GE almost entirely.

According to Isshiki (1964), GVTE varied as a function of vocal intensity (I) of an adult male, ranging from $0.9 \times 10^{-4}$ to $4.0 \times 10^{-4}$ for a low fundamental frequency, from $0.7 \times 10^{-4}$ to $14.0 \times 10^{-4}$ for a medium fundamental frequency, and from $0.3 \times 10^{-4}$ to $1.7 \times 10^{-4}$ for a high fundamental frequency.

## 2. Airflow-Intensity Profile

Saito (1977) reported the usefulness of airflow-intensity profile in evaluating the efficiency of phonation. With the use of a simultaneous recording system of the airflow rate and the vocal intensity, he presented a graphic demonstration in which the airflow rate is drawn in the upward direction while the intensity is in the downward direction (Fig. 7.7). The fundamental frequency level is also represented simultaneously on the same chart.

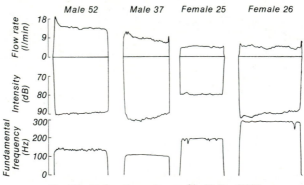

Fig. 7.7. Airflow-intensity profile (Saito, 1977)

## 3. Ratio of rms Value of AC Component to Mean Volume Velocity (DC Component)

With the use of a hot-wire flow meter, Isshiki (1977) measured the ratio of rms value of AC component of the volume velocity to mean volume velocity (Fig. 7.8). He named this ratio the "efficiency of voice". It is expressed as the following two formulae provided the glottal waveform is assumed to be triangular, and the glottal closure is incomplete.

$$\text{Efficiency of voice} = \frac{1}{\sqrt{3}}\left(\frac{1-x}{1+x}\right) \tag{4}$$

where,

$$x = \frac{\text{minimum glottal width (c in Figure 8)}}{\text{maximum glottal width (d in Figure 8)}} \tag{5}$$

For the vibration with a complete glottal closure, Flanagan (1958) calculated the value as shown below:

$$E = \sqrt{\frac{4-3q}{3q}} \tag{6}$$

$$\text{where } q = OQ = \frac{\text{time interval of open phase}}{\text{time interval of entire cycle}}$$

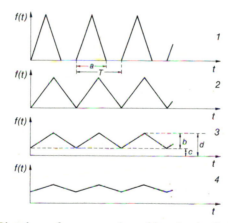

Fig. 7.8. Glottal waveforms approximated by triangles (Isshiki, 1977)

# References

Böhme, G., Hecker, G. (1970): Gerontologische Untersuchungen über Stimmumfang und Sprechstimmlage. Folia Phoniat. *22*, 176–184.

Coleman, R. F., Mabis, J. H., Hinson, J. K. (1977): Fundamental frequency-sound pressure level profiles of adult male and female voices. J. Sp. Hear. Res. *20*, 197–204.

Damsté, H. (1970): The phonetogram. Pract. ORL. *32*, 185–187.

Flanagan, J. L. (1958): Some properties of the glottal sound source. J. Sp. Hear. Res. *1*, 99—116.

Hayashi, Y. (1940): Lecture on voice and speech disorders, Part 7. Pract. Otol. (Kyoto) *34*, 210—214.

Hirano, M., Koike, Y., von Leden, H. (1968): Maximum phonation time and air usage during phonation. Clinical study. Folia Phoniat. *20*, 185—201.

Hollien, H., Dew, D., Philips, P. (1971): Phonation frequency ranges of adults. J. Sp. Hear. Res. *14*, 755—760.

Hollien, H., Shipp, T. (1972): Speaking fundamental frequency and chronologic age in males. J. Sp. Hear. Res. *15*, 155—159.

Ihda, T. (1940): Vocal range of Japanese. Fukuoka Med. J. *33*, 229—292.

Isshiki, N. (1964): Regulatory mechanism of voice intensity variation. J. Sp. Hear. Res. *7*, 17—29.

Isshiki, N. (1977): Functional surgery of the larynx. Dept. Otolaryngol., Kyoto Univ.

Isshiki, N., Okamura, H., Horimoto, M. (1967): Maximum phonation time and air flow rate during phonation: Simple clinical tests for vocal function. Ann. Otol. *76*, 998—1007.

Komiyama, S. (1972): Phonogram. A new method evaluating voice characteristics. Otologia (Fukuoka) *18*, 428—440.

Nishikawa, T. (1962): Study on the relationship between the voice and the states of the vocal cord. J. Otolaryngol. Jpn. *65*, 545—575.

Nishiyama, A. (1969): The range of voice in musical scale and the scale in conversational voice. Otolaryngol. (Tokyo) *41*, 877—880.

Ptacek, P. H., Sander, E. K. (1963): Maximum duration of phonation. J. Sp. Hear. Dis. *28*, 171—182.

Saito, S. (1977): Phonosurgery. Basic study on the mechanism of phonation and endolaryngeal microsurgery. Otologia (Fukuoka) *23*, 171—384.

Sawashima, M. (1966): Measurement of maximum phonation time. Jpn. J. Logoped. Phoniat. *7*, 23—28.

Sawashima, M. (1968): Clinical aspects of voice disorders. Jpn. J. Logoped. Phoniat. *9*, 9—14.

Schultz-Coulon, H. J. (1975): Bestimmung und Beurteilung der individuellen mittleren Sprechstimmlage. Experimentelle Studie. Folia Phoniat. *27*, 375—386.

Shigemori, Y. (1977): Some tests related to the air usage during phonation. Clinical investigations. Otologia (Fukuoka) *23*, 138—166.

Suzuki, T. (1944): Investigations of expiratory air volume during phonation. Tohoku Med. J. *34*, 93 to 104.

van Oordt, H. W. A., Drost, H. A. (1963): Development of the frequency range of the voice in children. Folia Phoniat. *15*, 289—298.

Yanagihara, N., Koike, Y., von Leden, H. (1966): Phonation and respiration. Function study in normal subjects. Folia Phoniat. *18*, 323—340.

# Subject Index

# Disorders
# of Human Communication

Edited by

**Godfrey E. Arnold,** Jackson, Miss., USA
**Fritz Winckel,** Berlin (West)
**Barry D. Wyke,** London, Great Britain

Volume 1
### Hearing: Its Function and Dysfunction
By **Earl D. Schubert**
1980. 86 figures. X, 184 pages.
ISBN 3-211-81579-1

Volume 2
### Clinical Aspects of Dysphasia
By **Martin L. Albert, Harold Goodglass,
Nancy A. Helm, Alan B. Rubens,
and Michael P. Alexander**
1981. 12 figures. XI, 194 pages.
ISBN 3-211-81617-8

Volume 3
### Clinical Linguistics
By **David Crystal**
1981. 3 figures. XII, 228 pages.
ISBN 3-211-81622-4

Volume 4
### Voice, Speech,
### and Language in the Child:
### Development and Disorder
By **John A. M. Martin**
1981. 43 figures. XVI, 210 pages.
ISBN 3-211-81629-1

Further volumes are in preparation
Prices are subject to change without notice

**Springer-Verlag
Wien
New York**

# Breathing, Speech, and Song

By **Donald F. Proctor,** M. D., The Johns Hopkins University,
School of Medicine and School of Hygiene and
Public Health, Baltimore, Md., USA

1980. 70 figures. XI, 176 pages.
ISBN 3-211-81580-5

BREATHING, SPEECH, AND SONG is written by a physician
whose career has included physiological research, the
study and practice of singing, and 42 years in the practice
of otolaryngology. Its contents are of interest to the
laryngologist and physiologist while, at the same time,
being intelligible to the teacher and student of the human
voice. It is profusely illustrated and carefully indexed. In
addition to a clear description of the normal structure and
function of the organs of breathing and phonation,
chapters deal with the art of effective speaking and singing,
care of the professional voice, and detection and correction
of vocal disabilities. Although its main theme is the role
of proper breathing in speech and song, it includes a
discussion of many of the factors essential to those for
whom the voice plays a central role in their professional
lives. No other book covers these subjects so clearly and
authoritatively.

Prices are subject to change without notice

**Springer-Verlag Wien New York**